MW01528828

Elimination Diet 101

A cookbook and how-to guide with helpful advice and 80 easy, quick and delicious recipes to test for food allergies and sensitivities

by
Jennifer Vasché Lehner

Text copyright © 2014 by Jennifer Vasché Lehner

Photographs copyright © Erin Seyfried

Design by Christine Williams

Edited by Mike Lehner

Printed and bound in the United States of America. All rights reserved. No part of this book may be reproduced or transmitted in any form or by any electronic or mechanical means including photocopying, microfilming, and recording, or by any information storage and retrieval systems without permission in writing from the publisher, except by a reviewer, who may quote brief passages in a review. Published by Jennifer Lehner, Mountain View, CA. EliminationDiet101@gmail.com.

Current Printing (last digit)

10 9 8 7 6 5 4 3 2

ISBN-13: 978-0-9885624-0-0

www.facebook.com/EliminationDiet101

Information found in this book, whether provided by Elimination Diet 101, its contributors, licensors or users, is for informational purposes only and is not intended to be a substitute for professional medical or dietary treatment. Every person is unique and a diet should reflect that. Always consult with your physician or a qualified health care provider before deciding on your diet.

Acknowledgements

If you enjoy this book, it is in no small part due to the fabulous group of people who inspired, shaped, and edited it. *Elimination Diet 101* truly represents the time, enthusiasm, and generous help they gave, and I would love for you to know who they are and how much I appreciate them. My heartfelt gratitude goes to:

My amazing husband Mike, for...everything. Six years ago someone had the audacious idea to write this book. I honestly don't remember if it was him or me, but that's a sign of how integral he's been to the entire process. Had he not cheerfully taken on so much of what I normally do in order to allow me the time to research, test and cook recipes, and write to my heart's content, this book would never have happened. His faith in my ability to complete a project of such magnitude is only slightly more remarkable than the 10 round-trip flights he took with our son to give me "recipe weekends" alone and the countless hours he devoted to the unloved but vital task of editing. He never once complained or allowed anything but supportive words to escape his lips. For always encouraging me when the task felt too great and continuing to love me when I was so completely absorbed in my own work, I am eternally grateful.

My loving parents, Janet and David, who have supported every endeavor I've ever undertaken. Looking back on my childhood, it's clear just how instrumental those healthy family dinners were that we shared every night! No matter where I go or what I do, I'm always my parents' daughter and I hope that this book makes them proud.

My wonderful in-laws, Pam and Chris, who have been such enthusiastic cheerleaders of the book, but more importantly, of me in general. I am so grateful for their support and for encouraging me to be confident in myself and my own talents. Oh, and also for their eagle eyes – readers will never know how many typos they didn't have to suffer through thanks to their editing efforts.

Christine Williams, my skilled designer, who stepped up at "crunch time" and so flawlessly translated my vision onto paper. Her design skills and many sensible suggestions regarding text, format, and flow vastly improved the presentation of this book – readers will benefit from her great work.

Erin Seyfried, whose photographic talents captured each recipe in such appetizing fashion. I am incredibly grateful for her support, steady hand, and long hours working side-by-side.

Kelly Morrow and Dr. Todd Born, who encouraged me to move forward with this book when it was still just a wishful concept. Both conducted thorough reviews, verified recipes for accuracy, and provided insightful comments that added great value and depth to the final draft. I am so thankful to be able to incorporate into this book some of the knowledge and wisdom they have gained in their many years of naturopathic experience. I am honored by the time they have invested and I hope that this book is a valuable resource for their patients.

And finally, my little Luke, whose laughter and smile puts everything in perspective. I can't say that he made this project easier, but he certainly does make me a better person every day and I love him so much. All this cookbook stuff is fabulous, but being Luke's mom is what fills my heart with joy.

It "only" took four years for this book to reach fruition and each of these lovely people was invaluable to me along that journey. We made it! Thank you all, so very much!

Table of Contents

Introduction   7-22

   The Basics   9
   Step By Step   12
   Tips & Tricks   14
   Table 1: Foods to Include & Exclude   20
   Table 2: Challenge Phase Schedule   21
   Table 3: Food Challenge Response Chart   22

Breakfast   23-27

   Go Nuts Smoothie   24
   The Hulk Smoothie   24
   Turkey Apple Breakfast Sausage   25
   Pumpkin Pie Quinoa Bake   26
   Millet, Rice & Quinoa Cereal   27

Soups & Salads   29-40

   Chinese Chicken Salad   30
   Salad Nicoise   31
   Southwestern Quinoa Salad   32
   Strawberry Spinach Salad   33
   Pear Harvest Salad   34
   Chicken & Pasta Broth   35
   Curried Vegetable Soup   37
   Butternut Squash Soup   38
   Black Bean Brew   39
   Cauliflower Bisque   40

Poultry & Meats   41-53

   Smothered Chicken   42
   Chicken Packets   43
   Turkey Cutlets with Blackberry Sauce   44
   Chicken Provence   45
   Roasted Cornish Game Hens   46

Tuscan BBQ Chicken	47
Turkey Burgers with Cranberry Sauce	48
Chicken Sausage Patties	49
Roasted Leg of Lamb	50
Fennel Pork Loin with Pears	51
Pistachio Pesto	52
Tropical Burger	53

Fish & Seafood — 55-60

Soba Noodle Salmon	56
Curried Shrimp with Rice	57
Pasta & Shrimp Packets	58
1-2-3 Salmon	59
Grilled Mahi-Mahi with Avocado-Melon Salsa	60

Pasta, Rice & Grains — 61-70

Creamy Avocado Pasta	62
Turkey Bolognese	63
Poor Man's Pesto	64
Roasted Butternut Squash & Shallots Pasta	65
Pea & Tuna Pasta Salad	66
Wild Rice a la California	67
Asparagus Risotto	68
Tri-Grain Pilaf	68
Creamy Rice & Spinach Casserole	69
Brown Rice & Bean Salad	70

Vegetables — 71-79

Lentils with Spinach	72
Roasted Brussels Sprouts	73
Wilted Lettuce & Peas	73
Winter Squash & Black Bean Saute	74
Roasted Beets	75
Broccoli Quinoa Pilaf	76
Millet & Cauliflower "Mashed Potatoes"	77
Spaghetti Squash with Mushrooms & Herbs	78
Roasted Acorn Squash	79

Snacks   81-85

Chips & Guacamole   82
Crispy Kale Chips   83
Power Balls   84
Hummus   85
Roasted Sweet Potato Wedges   86
Peanut Dipping Sauce   86

Desserts   87-91

Carob Mousse   88
Pear Compote   89
Banana Ice Cream   89
Rice Crispy Crunchies   90
Autumn Spice Latte   91

Challenge Phase   93-111

Lavender Lemonade   94
Coconut Lime Chicken   95
Grapefruit Brulee   96
Warm Chicken Citrus Salad   97
Roasted Corn on the Cob   98
Sweet Potato & Goat Cheese Bruschetta   99
Yogurt Medley   100
Eggs Anemone   101
Apple Pie Crockpot Oatmeal   102
Rye & Seed Crackers   103
Barley & Rice Pilaf   104
Chicken & Bulgar Pilaf   105
Sweet Potato Chicken Quesadilla   106
Roasted Eggplant Dip   107
Broccoli with Fennel & Red Bell Pepper   108
Seared Tuna with Garlic, Tomatoes & Herbs   109
Creamy Mashed Potatoes   110
Chicken Teriyaki Meatball Saute   111

About the Author   113

Introduction

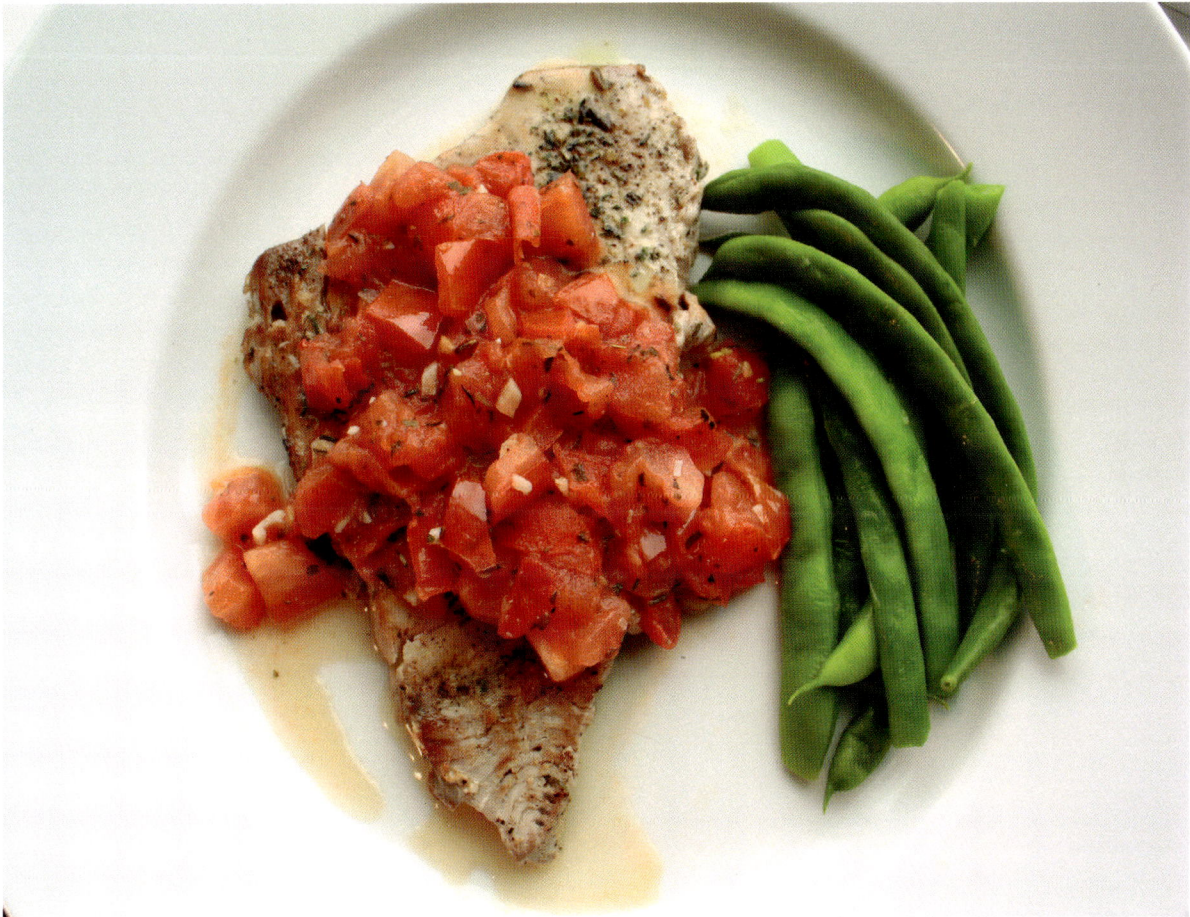

Seared Tuna with Garlic, Tomatoes & Herbs

INTRODUCTION

I'm so happy that you discovered the Elimination Diet and are ready to give it a try, and I'm even happier that you found my book! Why? Because I wrote it for **you**! I know firsthand that new journeys - particularly this one - can seem overwhelming at first, and I want to support you and reassure you that you can do this!

Every body is unique and our stories are all different, but we have found ourselves at the same place. We are in pain, we are uncomfortable, we may have been to countless medical appointments, tried weird medications, and still haven't found a solution. We are frustrated and know that something isn't quite right, but we don't know exactly what it is, and we want to feel better.

The vision for this book emerged 6 years ago when I was suffering from explosive skin rashes and intense body aches without any significant sign of serious illness or cause. I was poked, examined, x-rayed, and CT-scanned to exhaustion by multiple doctors of various specialties, only to be told that there was nothing "physically wrong" with me except for a mild case of psoriasis.

I trusted my doctors, but I knew deep down that they were wrong. I wasn't sure where to go next or what else to do, and I thought I had exhausted all of my options.

Then a good friend recommended that I visit a naturopathic doctor (ND). I had no idea what an ND was or what they did, but the recent psoriasis diagnosis had me very concerned about the prescribed lifetime of intensive steroid treatments that lay before me. After my first round of steroid treatment, I knew that I didn't want to continue exposing my body to those hormones - there must be another way, a better way....

At the first appointment, the ND recommended that I do the Elimination Diet to see if food sensitivities might be causing my symptoms. My first reaction was total surprise - it had never occurred to me, nor been suggested to me, that food (?!) might be the problem. My second reaction was mild devastation - I love food and, next to growing it, cooking it and eating it are my greatest passions. The ND gave me a small handbook of information about what not to eat along with a few sample recipes, asked me to make a follow-up appointment for the next month, and sent me on my way.

Flipping though the handbook on the bus ride home, I panicked - no wheat, eggs, dairy, tomatoes, potatoes, citrus, soy, sugar? What exactly _am_ I going to be able to eat? Will my husband, Mike, be willing to eat the same food as me, or will I have to cook two separate meals every evening? The handbook's recipes looked interesting, but there wasn't much variety. They required a lot of prep time and exotic ingredients that I was unable to realistically handle while working full-time. **_Can I actually do the Elimination Diet?_**, I asked myself.

I jumped off the bus and ran home, headed straight for the kitchen, and pulled my big binder of favorite recipes off the shelf. I spent the next several hours sifting through them to find Elimination Diet-friendly recipes and recipes that could be modified to be diet-friendly.

The result was a HUGE stack of quick, easy, and delicious recipes that gave me the confidence to commit to the Elimination Diet - even Mike agreed to join me on the journey, since it didn't seem like too much sacrifice to eat a lot of the same meals we were already eating. Excellent! I now had a rock-solid plan and the necessary tools to blast through the Elimination Diet - or so I thought.

Day 1 of the Elimination Diet was exciting and energetic. Day 2 was good, and Day 3 was OK. By Day 4, though, I was ready to throw in the towel. It turns out that I had accidentally been eating rice bread made with some egg whites. I had the worst headache of my life and a friend wanted Mike and I to come over for dinner that weekend - she was going to make her award-winning lasagna (try asking someone to modify a dish primarily composed of pasta, cheese, and tomato sauce to meet Elimination Diet requirements and they will not be pleased!).

It was a bad day for sure, but made more so because I wasn't prepared for all of these unhappy surprises. No one told me what it would actually feel like to do the Elimination Diet, and I was not a happy camper!

I took a few days off from the Diet to regroup and think carefully about what was really before me. How could I avoid accidentally eating prohibited foods? How could I still have a social life without completely eliminating food from the occasion? When was my headache going to go away? Would I have to put my real life "on-hold" and could I afford to do that for several months to do the Elimination Diet? I spent hours searching articles online, reading blogs and medical journals, and consulting my personal calendar - and then I developed a realistic game plan.

I started over, now empowered with more preparation about how to navigate life while staying true to the Elimination Diet. Mike and I breezed through the Elimination Phase for the next month. Next was the Challenge Phase - the fun part! After weeks of carefully adding foods back, I was surprised to learn that I have a wheat sensitivity. Of course, looking back over the past few years it all makes sense, but hindsight is 20/20! I got back to my normal life (just minus bread) and months later - surprise, surprise - my psoriasis and body pains cleared up completely. The Elimination Diet worked!

Friends and co-workers who learned of my experience began asking questions and wanting to try the diet, so I began bundling recipes and jotting down practical advice to share with them...this book began writing itself long before I knew I was going to write it.

I've been where you are right now. I was nervous about committing to the Elimination Diet, I was worried about my quality of life during the process, and I was baffled by what I was going

to eat. I won't lie, it was difficult - but only because I wasn't initially prepared for what was really involved and I didn't have the information I needed to meet those unexpected challenges. I had to do my own research, develop my own recipes, and seek out guidance from those who had come before me. In short, I didn't have a resource like this book to help me. And that's really why I've written this book. I want *you* to have an easy, delicious, and successful Elimination Diet experience - the recipes I've developed and the lessons I've learned, all shared in this book, will help you do just that.

My greatest hope is that this book will help you easily navigate through the Elimination Diet, enjoy the process, and emerge from that journey with the answers you need to heal yourself!

THE BASICS: Elimination Diet 101

Before setting out on the Elimination Diet, it's important to understand exactly what it is - the philosophy, the process, and logistics - so that you're empowered with the information you need to have an enjoyable and successful experience....

What is the Elimination Diet?

As the name implies, this diet is designed to identify food intolerances and sensitivities by temporarily eliminating foods from our diet that are known to frequently cause symptoms, and then systematically reintroducing them to observe for a reaction.

The Elimination Diet is divided into two phases - the *Elimination Phase* and the *Challenge Phase*. The Elimination Phase begins by eliminating all suspect foods (there are a lot of them!) from your diet for a period of time that is long enough to allow your body to fully process and eliminate them, about 2-4 weeks. If one or more of the eliminated foods is causing your symptoms, those symptoms should subside or disappear by the end of this period. This leads to the Challenge Phase. Those eliminated foods are systematically added back into your diet, one at a time, to test for a reaction. If a reaction is observed, it can then be easily determined which food has caused your symptoms to return.

Reactions can range from mild to intense, but most are caused by a food intolerance or sensitivity rather than a true food allergy. A food intolerance or sensitivity can produce some of the same signs and symptoms as a true food allergy, so people often confuse them. However, it is important to recognize the difference because one means not being able to eat *any* amount of a particular food while the others mean just making judicious decisions about when and how much of a food to eat:

- A food **allergy** causes an immediate immune system response that can affect numerous organs in the body. The body's immune system normally defends against potentially harmful substances, but sometimes an immune response is triggered by a substance that is generally harmless - like a specific food. The immune response can produce a range of reactions, sometimes severe or life-threatening like anaphylaxis (when the throat swells shut and blood pressure drops). Some of the most common life threatening food allergies are peanuts, tree nuts, and shellfish. True food allergies are much less common than intolerances or sensitivities.

- A food **intolerance** can share some of the symptoms of food allergies, but is a digestive incompatibility rather than an immune system response. People with food intolerances are not able to digest certain foods, either because their body may lack a necessary digestive enzyme or because there may be a food component that a person does not digest well for genetic or other reasons. Food intolerances can cause discomfort but are not life-threatening. Some of the most

common food intolerances are lactose (milk sugar), fructose (fruit sugar) and sorbitol (sugar alcohol).

- A food **sensitivity** is a mild allergy that causes a mild immune system response which often appears gradually within hours to days after exposure. The symptoms are less serious and intense than a true food allergy. Examples include sore joints, diarrhea, emotional imbalance, and skin rashes.

Why do the Elimination Diet?

You're probably asking yourself "Is all this *really* necessary?" There are many good reasons to consider the Elimination Diet, even if you don't think you have a food intolerance or sensitivity.

Countless numbers of people suffer from food intolerances and sensitivities - often without being aware of it. According to current research, they can cause or contribute to a vast array of problems including:

- fatigue
- anxiety and depression
- insomnia
- joint pain
- food cravings
- nasal congestion and runny nose
- Irritable Bowel Syndrome (IBS)
- gas and bloating
- constipation and diarrhea
- abdominal pain and stomach cramps
- gallbladder disease
- high blood pressure
- acne and rashes
- eczema and psoriasis
- muscle aches
- migraines
- respiratory difficulty

Most of the above symptoms can have more than one contributor, but food is a relatively common yet frequently overlooked cause. Since many sensitivities and intolerances cannot be clearly identified using blood or skin tests, one of the least invasive and most effective ways to identify the foods which may be causing these symptoms is the Elimination Diet.

We're also less likely to associate food with the resulting symptoms when there's a delay or gradual appearance between eating and the symptoms occurring. People with a food intolerance or sensitivity may not experience symptoms unless they eat a large portion of the food or eat that food frequently. At times, symptoms may be delayed. For all these reasons, food intolerances and sensitivities are much harder to diagnose than food allergies. The Elimination Diet's process isolates problem foods so that you can reliably associate cause and effect.

The Elimination Diet can also jump start us out of "food ruts" and identify any lurking food addictions that may surface as cravings or withdrawal symptoms (coffee, anyone?!). Daily repetition of the same foods is thought to be a major contributor to the development of food sensitivities, and hopefully the process and the recipes in this cookbook encourage you to try and enjoy new foods.

Not surprisingly, many people experience improvement in various symptoms when following the Elimination Diet. If you stop eating refined sugar and white flour, you'll generally wind up cutting out most processed foods, which tend to be high in calorie content and low in nutritive value. Within a few weeks of replacing processed foods with fresh ones, it shouldn't be a surprise if you start to feel better too!

Who should do the Elimination Diet?

Because adverse food reactions can contribute to several medical conditions, identifying and eliminating any foods that cause these reactions can be very helpful for most people. Elimination Dieters may experience uncomfortable symptoms caused by detoxification (including headache, muscle pains, or fatigue) during the first week of the Diet, though

these symptoms usually disappear within seven days. When offending foods are reintroduced into the diet during the Challenge Phase, Elimination Dieters can experience mild to severe reactions to food, so it is important to complete the Elimination Diet only under the advice and supervision of a health care provider.

Who should NOT do the Elimination Diet?

Individuals with respiratory reactions (such as asthma, bronchitis, respiratory distress syndrome, chronic obstructive pulmonary disease or emphysema) or any family or personal history of anaphylaxis (a severe whole-body allergic reaction) should not do the Elimination Diet, at least not without direct medical supervision, as it could be life-threatening.

People who suspect gluten sensitivity, have a history of anemia, or have a family history of celiac disease should be screened for celiac disease as it is difficult to properly diagnose after long-term elimination. Celiac disease is an autoimmune disease that may affect as many as 1 in 133 people in the U.S. The most common symptoms include diarrhea, constipation, skin rash, anemia, and poor growth in childhood.

Individuals with eating disorders, even in their past, should only attempt the Elimination Diet if their health care provider is confident that it will not pose a risk.

Which foods can I eat during the Elimination Diet?

Because there are so many potentially allergenic/sensitive foods that can cause symptoms, there is an extensive list of food and food groups that you'll need to steer clear of during the Elimination Phase of the diet and the majority of the Challenge Phase. The good news is that there's an even more extensive list of allowed foods that you *can* enjoy! Table 1 lists the foods that you can and cannot eat, and as you progress through the Diet it will become second nature. In the beginning, though, it's definitely helpful to have Table 1 at your fingertips to help with recipe planning and dining out options.

The foods listed in Table 1 are general guidelines, but you'll want to work with your health care provider to assess whether any additional foods should also be excluded. You might want to keep a diet journal for a week or so before beginning the Elimination Diet, listing the foods you eat and keeping track of the symptoms you have throughout the day. It's also helpful to ask yourself the following questions:

- What foods do I eat most often?
- What foods do I crave?
- What foods do I eat to "comfort myself"?
- What foods would I have trouble giving up?

Often, these are the very foods that are most important to eliminate during the Elimination Diet! Based on your symptoms, current diet, and answers to the above questions, your health care provider may want to exclude additional items such as sulfites, salicylates, fermented products, or other foods that promote yeast overgrowth. If so, you'll need to review the recipes in this book to ensure that they still meet your dieting needs.

How Do I Use This Book?

Just as the Elimination Diet is divided into two simple phases, this cookbook is divided into two sections that address each of those phases: the *Elimination Phase* section and the *Challenge Phase* section. In the Elimination Phase section, you'll find recipes that use only Elimination Diet-allowed foods (see Table 1 for those allowed foods). There are quite a few recipes to choose from, divided into color-coded sections: Breakfast, Soups & Salads, Poultry & Meats, Fish & Seafood, Pasta, Rice & Grains, Vegetables, Snacks, and Desserts (yes, you *can* have dessert on the Elimination Diet).

In the Challenge Phase section, you'll find one recipe for each food or food group that will be added back into your diet during the Challenge Phase of the Elimination Diet. These recipes will each be used once during the Elimination Diet (on the day that you are testing for that particular food), but of course you can enjoy them again after you've completed the entire Elimination Diet process! If you prefer to test using only the pure form of each food then you don't need to prepare these recipes, but they are so delicious that I think you'd be missing out if you skipped them. Table 2 outlines a suggested schedule of which foods to challenge and in which order.

All of the recipes in this book have been thoroughly reviewed for their adherence to the Elimination Diet regimen and vetted in my family's kitchen - only the tastiest, easiest, and least expensive have made the cut. I think you'll be pleased, and find these recipes to be the keys to a successful and enjoyable Elimination Diet experience.

STEP BY STEP: Doing the Elimination Diet

The Elimination Diet is divided into two simple phases - the *Elimination Phase* and the *Challenge Phase*.

STEP 1: Elimination Phase

During the Elimination Phase, you should completely avoid all foods known to cause reactions for 2-4 weeks. During this time, you'll enjoy foods that are generally considered non-reactive, allowing your body time to recover and symptoms to clear. Table 1 outlines the various food and food groups that are allowed and not allowed during this phase - follow this list and you're well on your way to a successful Elimination Diet journey. All of the recipes in the *Elimination Phase* section of this cookbook are allowed throughout this process, as they contain none of the ingredients that need to be avoided. You'll want to review this list with your health provider to ensure that you will be avoiding all the foods that they recommend. Sometimes, you'll need to transfer Elimination Diet-allowed food from the "Include" to "Exclude" side of the list if there are additional foods or food groups beyond the traditional Elimination Diet roster that might be of concern.

Please note that cheating is not allowed! Because any exposure can cause a reaction, cheating here and there will completely negate the purpose of the Elimination Diet. Your symptoms may not subside and you will not be able to move on to the Challenge Phase testing.

If you complete the Elimination Phase with no reduction in your symptoms, this does not mean that the Diet was unsuccessful. In fact, quite the opposite - you now know that the foods you removed probably aren't a primary cause of your symptoms. This is very useful information to have as you and your doctor explore the next steps in identifying the underlying cause of your health concerns, including whether or not to try the Elimination Diet again with a different combination of foods. On the other hand, some people do not notice much of anything on the Elimination Phase but are still able to identify some food-related issues during the Challenge Phase. If you are unsure about continuing on to the Challenge Phase, consult with your health care provider.

STEP 2: Challenge Phase

If your symptoms improve after completing 2-4 weeks of the Elimination Phase, you're ready to move on to the Challenge Phase. During this next phase, you'll start "challenging" your body with the eliminated foods, one food group at a time, once every three days (it can take up to three days to be sure that any delayed reactions have time to surface). If a reaction does occur within this window, you'll be able to confidently associate it with this food. As you introduce new challenge foods, you should record any response or symptoms that you experience (see Table 3).

Each recipe in the Challenge Phase section of this book is essentially an Elimination Phase recipe (meeting all the standards of allowed foods) with the singular addition of one new challenge item. When talking about the Challenge Phase, I often refer to these recipes as "Plus 1s." That helps reinforce the concept that this phase is about adding back in just one food at a time and that when you're not testing for a food you need to keep eating the Elimination Phase foods.

You should work with your health care provider to determine the order in which you will challenge foods. Standard procedure is to first challenge those foods that you *least* suspect to be problematic and work your way up to those foods that you do suspect are causing symptoms. That way you don't unnecessarily experience any potential reactions early on and have to start the whole process over to let symptoms subside. Table 2 suggests a generalized schedule for which foods to challenge and in what order. The process for the Challenge Phase is as follows:

1. Begin the Challenge Phase after completing 2-4 weeks of the Elimination Phase. If your symptoms have not improved in that time, talk with your health care provider about whether or not to try it again with a different combination of foods. If your symptoms did improve during the Elimination Phase, continue to the Challenge Phase.

2. On Day 1 of the Challenge Phase, consume the selected challenge food 2-3 times throughout the day. For at least one exposure, try to choose a "pure" form of the food (fresh squeezed lemon juice to test for lemons, for example). For the other exposure, you may use this book's Challenge Phase recipe for that corresponding food. For each exposure, make sure that you consume enough of that food for your digestive system to notice that it's there. For your other meals and snacks on Day 1, consume only allowed Elimination Phase food.

3. On Days 2 and 3, consume only allowed Elimination Phase food. Observe for any reaction and do not consume challenge foods on these days. Problem foods may not be immediately obvious since food sensitivities can go unnoticed for hours or even days after being digested.

4. If there is no reaction, introduce a new challenge food on Day 4 and repeat the process.

5. If a reaction does occur, stop consuming the challenge food. Record the results in Table 3. Return to Elimination Phase food for at three additional days, or more until the reaction subsides. Reactions typically subside within three days, but can sometimes take longer. **Caution:** If you have an immediate allergic reaction, such as throat swelling, seek medical care and avoid food challenges unless you are under direct medical supervision.

6. Return to the Challenge Phase schedule and introduce a new challenge food again on the fourth day and repeat the entire process.

7. Follow-up with your health care provider once all foods have been challenged. Review the results from the completed Table 3 and discuss next-steps for diet and nutrition planning based on the identified food sensitivities.

You'll notice in Table 2 that some foods have sub-categories (gluten, citrus, nightshades , etc.) that are challenged individually. For example, when testing for gluten during the Challenge Phase, you'll be testing each type of gluten grain separately (wheat, rye, barley, etc.). Why is this? Because our bodies are so wonderfully quirky and unique! For those with gluten intolerance, for example, some types of gluten might cause problems and others might not. You might do fine with rye, but not with wheat. It can be the same for nightshade vegetables and citrus - maybe you can tolerate mashed potatoes every day, but bell peppers put your stomach through the ringer. Thus, you'll need to isolate and thoroughly test separate foods

within the Challenge Phase categories in order to properly rule them out.

Some health care providers modify the Challenge Phase for their patients who can't commit to the full regimen. For example, patients may be asked to test only certain foods or just experiment with different grains, citrus fruits, etc., for the next few months or years without restricting their diet to Elimination Phase foods. Consult with your health care provider about any modifications they or you think should be made to your Elimination Diet experience. Many of you can expect to find at least one food that you're intolerant or sensitive to, even if you previously hadn't noticed any problems. Sensitivities can also range widely in their intensity and health implications, so some of you will now need to completely avoid that food while others can use this experience simply as a cautionary tale for overindulging, but not completely avoiding.

Far fewer of you will find that you are actually truly allergic to a food - but for those of you that do, count yourselves very lucky to have finally found out! Either way, the next step is to work closely with your doctor to investigate what is behind the sensitivity, intolerance, or allergy and develop a plan to address that food's role in your diet.

TIPS AND TRICKS: Advice for a successful Elimination Diet journey!

If you live in a bubble, your Elimination Diet experience (along with many other things in your life!) will be a cake-walk. But you don't, so it won't. You have a real life - family, friends, work, social events, grocery shopping - and depending on your lifestyle and commitments, the Elimination Diet will probably put a proverbial cramp in your style. There's no need to become a dieting martyr, but some practical adjustments will be required. Fortunately, these adjustments are temporary and can be a great excuse to try new things!

I honestly believe that the practical, day-to-day execution of the diet can be more challenging than the dietary instructions themselves. Whether you are Elimination Dieting or not, life marches on, and I had to learn for myself how to create harmony. Hopefully you can adopt some lessons from my experiences to better enjoy your own Elimination Diet journey!

Double Duty

Perhaps the most important feature of the recipes in this book is that, as all good recipes should be, they are delicious, quick, and inexpensive. All this adds up to a repertoire of food that will please both you and any lucky folks with whom you are dining. Why relegate oneself to cooking multiple dinners when an Elimination Diet recipe is at least as good as what otherwise would have been prepared?

My paramount concern when presented with the concept of the Elimination Diet was that I would have to cook separate meals for myself and my husband. With all the dietary restrictions, how could I possibly ask him to suffer through the month eating the same meals as me? However, I'm a busy mom, I work full-time outside the home, and I have taken responsibility for preparing three meals a day for my family. So, I'm certainly not interested or even available to be cooking personalized meals for everyone - even for myself!

The recipes that I collected and cooked throughout the Elimination Diet - the same recipes that I am sharing in this book - put that concern to rest as both my husband and I marched through the month well fed and satisfied, sharing the same Elimination Diet meals. (That doesn't mean that he didn't slip out on his own for the occasional burger or fish 'n' chips when he wanted to!) To ensure that everyone will be happy eating together, each

of the offerings in this book meets my three "non-negotiables" for a good recipe:

1. **DELICIOUS** enough to serve my in-laws. Who *doesn't* want to impress their guests with a scrumptious home-made spread? Each of the recipes in this book has received multiple compliments and requests for copies. What this means is that those with whom you regularly dine will be unsuspecting and more than happy to inadvertently join you in your Elimination Diet meal. I love you, Pam and Chris!

2. **QUICK** to prepare. My family starts circling the kitchen like vultures the minute I step in the door after work, so I need to be able to get dinner on the table pronto - yesterday isn't fast enough for my boys. Simple preparation, a short ingredients list of basic staples, and steps that can be taken the night before are essential to mimicking a line order chef and preventing my family from impatiently pounding their forks on the table.

3. **INEXPENSIVE** ingredients to buy. There's no greater thrill than throwing together a gourmet meal for pennies, and the happiness of my meal is often reduced when I've had to spend a lot of cash on expensive ingredients. There's certainly no reason that the Elimination Diet needs to break the bank. In fact, you're likely to save money by cooking at home if you're accustomed to eating out!

As long as the food is delicious and provides balanced nutrition, there's no reason the Elimination Diet needs to cause a lot of fuss and logistical nightmares.

Label Literacy

The surefire strategy for the Elimination Diet is to eat only allowed natural, whole foods served raw or gently cooked and seasoned with only natural salt, pepper, olive oil, herbs, or natural sweeteners. But what you DON'T eat is just as important. For your results to be successful, you have to avoid all potentially suspect foods and chemicals.

If you've read any food labels recently, you understand that deciphering exactly what is in your food is a confusing and frustrating task. Soy, corn, and gluten cooking products and additives go by many scary-sounding names (malodextrin! ascorbic acid!), and often appear as mystery ingredients in very small print buried deep in the ingredients list. This is legitimately annoying, and you will need to arm yourself with knowledge and patience to protect the integrity of your diet. It's hard enough to say "No!" to the *known* ingredients we can't eat on the diet - now we have to be worried about accidentally eating those hidden ingredients in our well-intentioned food choices!

The best advice, as mentioned above, is to eat as many whole natural foods as possible. It's pretty hard to get in trouble that way. Where we enter dangerous territory is in buying processed, packaged foods that advertise themselves as being "_____-free." As such, I really recommend a visit your local health food store that carries a wide variety of produce and natural food products. These stores employ very nice and knowledgeable people who will be only too happy to support your needs, give you a tour of the store, and advise which of their products you can utilize. The Elimination Diet process lasts a while, so I guarantee you'll find yourself in that store at some point anyway. Call ahead and schedule a visit, you'll be glad you did. It's a great way to mentally prepare for the Elimination Diet and get your fridge properly stocked for success.

Here are a couple quick pointers for navigating the grocery store aisles, though you'll probably need to do additional research on your own based on what your local health food store carries or what you find on your pantry shelves:

1. Stock up on allowed fresh fruits and vegetables that are certified organic and are in season. This should be the majority of what you'll be eating for the month. Fresh-frozen foods are good substitutes when fresh is unavailable or too expensive.

2. Some commercially-available poultry are injected with chemicals and are basted with corn starch, additives, and tenderizers. The label will usually state if a fresh chicken or turkey has not been treated.

3. Look for fresh fish, and avoid fillets treated with sulfites and other chemicals (such as farm raised fish).

4. Commercial salt and other seasonings often contain corn starch and chemicals. Purchase pure sea salt (which tastes much better anyway) and check the spice labels to makes sure they don't contain any unwanted ingredients.

5. Some commercially available nuts contain additives that are tossed in starch. Buy nuts in the shell (or fresh shelled with no processing), which are usually available at your local health food store. However, try to avoid purchasing nuts from the bulk bins because there can be cross-contamination among the bins and scoopers.

6. Drink only pure water (pure spring water, mineral water bottled in glass, or filtered water), not flavored.

7. Avoid most processed, smoked or cured meats (salami, bacon, sausage, etc.) - any surprise that there's a bunch of starches, sugar, and additives in there?

8. Check your vitamins! Many brands use dairy, soy, or gluten to help the medicine go down. Your doctor or local healthy food store can steer you towards Elimination Diet-friendly versions for the next 2-3 months.

This list is by no means comprehensive, but you get the idea. Just use your common sense and take the time to really read your labels. If you can't be bothered, stick to whole foods (though you will pay the price with limited meal options).

Dealing with Detox

The Elimination Diet is a natural detoxification process for your body. That's nice, but we also know what detox *really* means - withdrawal. It's true that cravings and withdrawal symptoms are common when embarking upon the Diet - after all, why wouldn't they be? Our bodies are sure to miss all the yummy addictive foods we eat, and sometimes Elimination Dieters can actually feel worse before they feel better. Typical complaints include nagging cravings, headaches, body aches, upset stomach, and lethargy...good times!

But seriously, the good news is that detox symptoms are usually limited to the first week. The even better news is that these symptoms often mean the diet is actually working! It's a paradox, but withdrawal and cravings themselves can be symptoms of food sensitivities - sometimes our favorite foods may be the very things that we're sensitive to. For me, it was wheat. For you, maybe cheese or eggs. Either way, the fact that your body is so desperate to have them probably means that something is suspicious!

The first week of the Elimination Diet can be truly irksome if you're detoxing, but there's a lot you can do to feel better. First and foremost, drink a lot of water! There's no faster way to flush the junk out of your system, and your skin will love you for it.

Another natural tool that can provide relief are essential oils. The plant compounds found in (therapeutic-grade) essential oils such as peppermint and lavender can often alleviate or eliminate fatigue, headaches, cravings, upset stomachs and skin breakouts – they can be used year-round throughout your life for many different ailments, but they seem particularly well-suited to addressing the common detox symptoms that so frequently occur with elimination diets. If you decide to add essential oils to your detox tool kit, please do your homework when selecting a brand – a lot of oils on the market (even those sold at health food stores that are labeled as "pure") are not really pure thera-peutic-grade and contain chemicals, additives, or are mostly made of water.

In those dark moments of temptation and cravings, it helps to remember that the Elimination Diet is a very *short-term* investment in your *long-term* future - a temporary inconvenience in exchange for a potential lifetime of good health. Not to mention that willpower is a muscle that grows stronger with exercise. Running in the opposite direction from the deli when you're dying for a tuna melt has a wonderful multiplying effect, as each act of positive choices reinforces your determination to carry on. And really, who wants to put in all the hard work of Week 1 only to blow the Diet on Week 2 and have to start over? If you're desperate, set a timer for 15 minutes and put that tempting treat out of sight. Studies show that cravings usually pass within 10 minutes, particularly if you can't see the object of your desire.

When all else fails, try going French. French women commonly cite distraction as a powerful tool in curbing their cravings and immediate culinary desires. For sure, distraction is a wonderful weapon when going into battle with your better-than-a-lover croissant craving. Naps, calling a long-lost friend, a short walk, or tackling your "honey-do" list can help, and they're all things you should really be making time for anyway!

The Elimination Diet may be a radical change for some of us, and each of our bodies will respond differently. While most Elimination Dieters experience both short- and long-term health benefits, the first week may be a bit rough and is usually the hardest. Abstaining from our traditional diet and favorite foods can be a challenge, but it's clearly worth it.

All You Need is Love...

I can't over-emphasize how important it is to surround yourself with positive support while on the Elimination Diet (let alone *all* the time!). Those friends and family with whom you regularly dine and socialize have the power to precipitate a Diet experience that is either really manageable or really oppressive. Food is an integral part of our daily existence, so having to adjust your menu also means having to adjust your life - this is much easier to achieve when the people around you are supportive! I'd recommend sitting down with your family or close friends to explain what the Elimination Diet is, how it works, and why you are doing it. It will help them understand that this is an important process in helping you achieve good health and well-being. The Elimination Diet is not some sort of egomaniacal, self-indulgent spa treatment, and the people who really care about you will cheer your efforts and gladly embrace the temporary inconveniences.

I was very fortunate, as Mike was eager to partner with me in brainstorming recipe ideas that we could eat together for dinner. He volunteered to limit his non-Diet food to outside the home or when I wasn't around - what a guy! We explained the Diet to friends with whom we regularly shared dinners and family whom we visit, so that everyone knew what to expect at mealtime. I was so reluctant and embarrassed to be making such a fuss about food, but everyone was actually very accepting and supportive! Think about it - for however much you don't want to dictate the menu to your dinner host, they also don't want to serve something you can't eat! Through the act of educating my friends about the Elimination Diet, I even inspired some of them to try it too. For me, the key was to invite my support net-work into the process by sharing information and providing suggestions about how they could best help me. The people who love you should and *do* want the best for you!

Dining In

It's possible, but dining out at restaurants is risky business for the Elimination Dieter. Though many restaurants offer allergen information for menu items, this information is not always complete or accurate. For example, did you know that certain commercial spice mixes contain cornstarch? That's probably not noted on the menu descriptions and, unless I can go back in the kitchen myself, I don't trust that the chef knows it either. And let's not even get started on salad dressings! It's also difficult to control for cross-contamination with non-Diet-allowed foods in a restaurant kitchen since equipment and cookware are often reused between orders.

Dining out should be avoided during the Elimination Phase in order to achieve reliable results - it's all too easy to accidentally eat a non-Diet-allowed food. If you do find yourself obligated to eat at a restaurant, you might be able to access their menus on-line before-hand or call ahead to select the best options. When in any doubt, play it safe and order a garden salad with olive oil dressing only - or bring your *own* dressing!

If your fridge is filled with take-out boxes, think of this as your big opportunity to clean it out, scrub it down (when was the last time you did that?!), and stock it with lovely green, organic produce. The best way to ensure that you are eating the right foods for the Elimination Diet is to prepare them yourself, not put your faith in the line chef at a 24-hour diner. Moreover, eating at home is cheaper, more nutritious, and can be just plain fun. It's befitting to honor the occasion and celebrate your meals - use fancy plates and linens, light candles, serve water in wine glasses, and play some music. The Elimination Diet is also a great opportunity to take a food safari - use this month as an excuse to work up the nerve to try some unusual new vegetable that you've always been curious about. Kohlrabi, anyone?

Get a life!

The Elimination Diet is not, I repeat, *not*, an excuse to stop living your life and having a good time at it! If you are a social nightlife creature, you'll just need to get a bit creative.

Your friends may need you to take the lead in crafting social opportunities that don't gravitate around restaurants and bars and food, which is surprisingly easy once you get the hang of it. Organize a game night, explore a new part of town or a park together, watch movies, check out a new band at the local coffee shop, or (like Mike and I did) join an evening kickball league or learn a new sport. These activities can be much more fun than eating lukewarm cheese fries in a smoky dive bar. If you do find yourself in a bar (some of us just seem to naturally gravitate toward them), order sparkling water in a martini glass and just let your imagination do the rest.

If you are invited to a dinner party, go! Just offer to bring an Elimination Diet-friendly side dish so you can be assured to have at least one item on your plate you can eat. Or better yet, offer to host the dinner party yourself so that *you* can plan the menu. Most Elimination Diet meals are so good your friends won't suspect a thing.

It goes without saying that holiday seasons aren't the most opportune time to initiate the Elimination Diet, so for your own sanity please try not to do so. I think I'd cry if I had to turn down a slice of my mother's pumpkin pie at Thanksgiving dinner. If you have the flexibility, check out your calendar for chunks of weeks that will present the fewest challenges for sticking to the diet. Starting the program a week before your wedding, for example, would not be a good choice. If you can reschedule events to clear a block of time, do that, particularly in the summer when fresh produce is bountiful, cheaper, and the general population tends to eat fresher, whole foods anyway.

It's all of these little choices and strategies that, when added up, mitigate the Elimination Diet's potential inconvenience and adverse impact on your daily life. The goal is to breeze through the process inspired and well-fed, not deprived. Remember, you are just eliminating some foods for a few weeks, not your whole life and happiness as you know it forever. If you're concerned that your lifestyle can't adjust and accommodate the Elimination Diet, I hope my advice convinces you that you can do it

flawlessly. With supportive friends and family, and armed with a good quality frying pan, the Elimination Diet will be a rewarding adventure that you will be glad you embarked upon.

Table 1: FOODS TO INCLUDE AND EXCLUDE

	INCLUDE	EXCLUDE
Fruits	Whole fruits (unsweetened, frozen, or water-packed), fruit juices (in small amounts)	All citrus fruits (orange, lemon, lime, grapefruit)
Vegetables	Fresh, raw, steamed, baked, roasted	Corn, canned vegetables, nightshades (tomato, potato, peppers, eggplant)
Dairy	Almond, rice, cashew, hemp, flax, hazelnut, and coconut milks	Eggs, milk, cheese, yogurt, butter, ice cream, non-dairy creamers, cottage cheese, cream cheese, kefir, casein, whey
Grains & Starch	Non-gluten grains (brown rice quinoa, millet, buckwheat, amaranth, teff, sorghum, mesquite, tapioca)	Wheat, corn, barley, bulgur, spelt, rye, oats, durum, semolina, emmer, faro
Legumes	Lentils, green beans, peas, dried beans (for example: chickpea, black, kidney, navy)	Peanuts, soy products (soy sauce, tofu, soy milk, soybean oil in processed foods)
Nuts & Seeds	Almonds, walnuts, pecans, sesame, cashews, nut and seed butters, pistachios, peanuts	All nuts and seeds are allowed
Animal Protein	Fish, chicken, turkey, lamb, wild game, beef, pork	Sausage, cold cuts, hot dogs, canned meat, eggs
Oils & Fats	Natural oils (olive, flax, coconut, walnut, sunflower)	Butter, margarine, shortening, mayonnaise, bottled salad dressings, canola (unless organic cold-pressed)
Beverages	Water, herbal tea, mineral water, coconut water	Coffee, tea, soda, alcohol, distilled water, all caffeinated beverage
Spices & Condiments	Salt, pepper, garlic, vinegar, tumeric, cinnamon, cumin, dill, ginger, oregano, basil, parsley, rosemary, thyme, turmeric, mustard, carob powder	Cayenne pepper, paprika, curry powder containing cayenne pepper, ketchup, relish, soy sauce, barbecue sauce, teriyaki, spice mixes with corn starch or additives, chocolate
Sweeteners (in small amounts)	Honey, maple syrup, brown rice syrup, Stevia	White or brown sugar, agave, corn syrup, Splenda, Equal, Nutrasweet, etc.

Table 2: CHALLENGE PHASE SCHEDULE

DAY	FOOD TO ADD
1	Lemon
4	Lime
7	Grapefruit
10	Orange
13	Corn
16	Soy
19	Eggs
22	Eggplant
25	Peppers
28	Tomato
31	Potato
34	Oats
37	Rye
40	Barley
43	Bulgur
46	Wheat
49	Goat milk
52	Cow milk
55	Coffee / Tea
58	Alcohol
61	Chocolate

Table 3: FOOD CHALLENGE RESPONSE CHART

Date	Food Introduced		Digestion/ Bowel Function	Joint/Muscle Aches	Headache/ Sinus, Congestion	Skin Changes (hives, rash, acne, itching, etc.)	Energy Level/ Fatigue	Other
	Time	Food						

Adapted from Bastyr Center for Natural Health

Breakfast

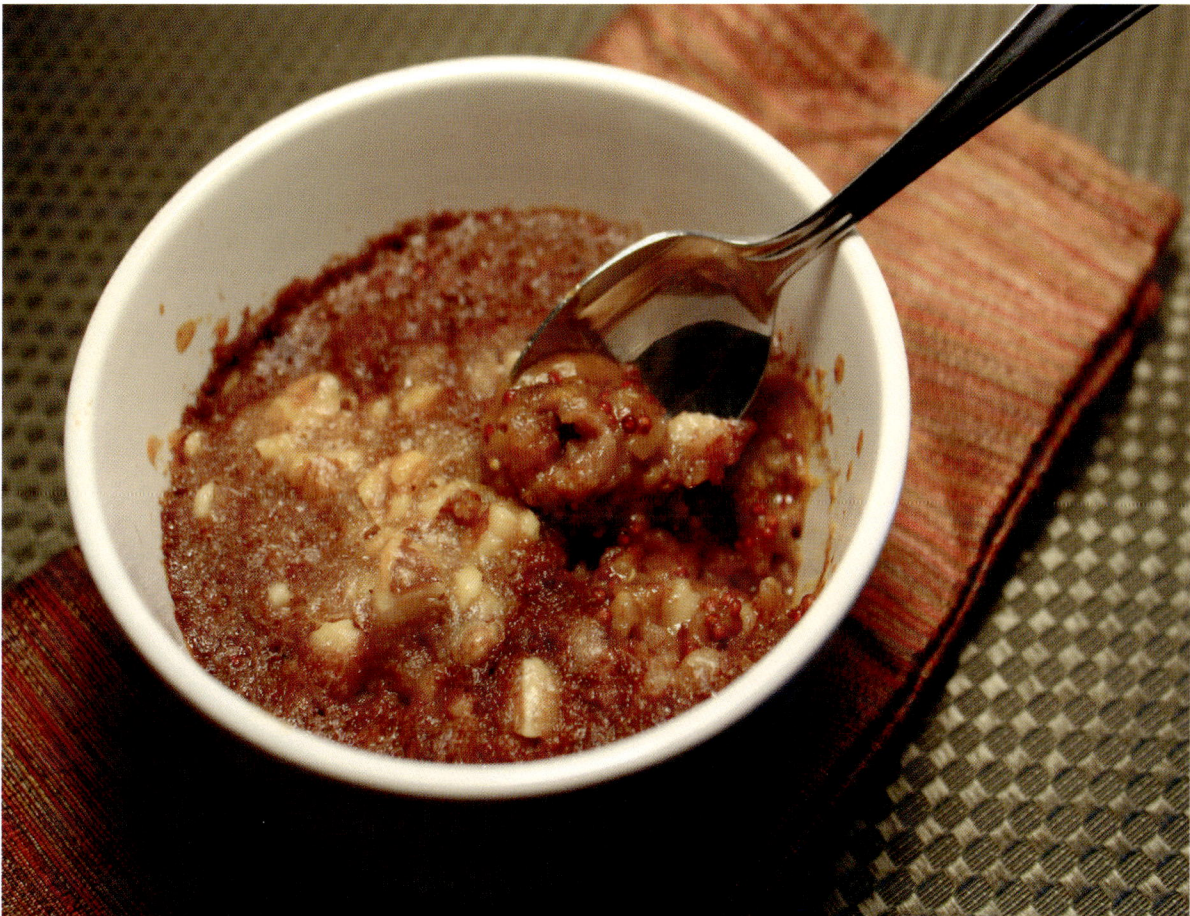

Pumpkin Pie Quinoa Bake

Go Nuts Smoothie

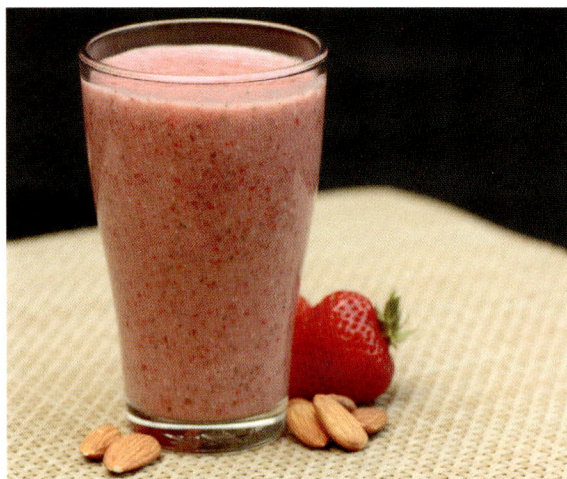

The addition of nuts to an otherwise basic fruit smoothie amps its nutritional quality with extra protein. Any fruit will do, but berries have phenomenal antioxidant properties that combat aging and disease. Organically-grown berries are plentiful and inexpensive when in season, but not so much in the winter – if you're doing the Elimination Diet during the winter months, it is best to choose frozen organic berries over imported produce that likely is doused in pesticides.

Serves 1

> 1/2 cup almond milk
> 1 cup strawberry, blueberry, blackberry or raspberry (fresh or frozen) or a mixture of each
> 1/2 banana, peeled or 1/2 apple, cored
> 3 Tablespoon walnuts or almonds, chopped
> 1/2 cup ice cubes
> 2 dates or two tablespoons agave
> 1 teaspoon vanilla (optional)
> 2 teaspoon slivered or sliced almonds

1. Put the first seven ingredients into the blender in the order listed.
2. Blend for 1 minute or until desired consistency is reached.
3. Pour smoothie into a tall glass and sprinkle with the almonds.

The Hulk Smoothie

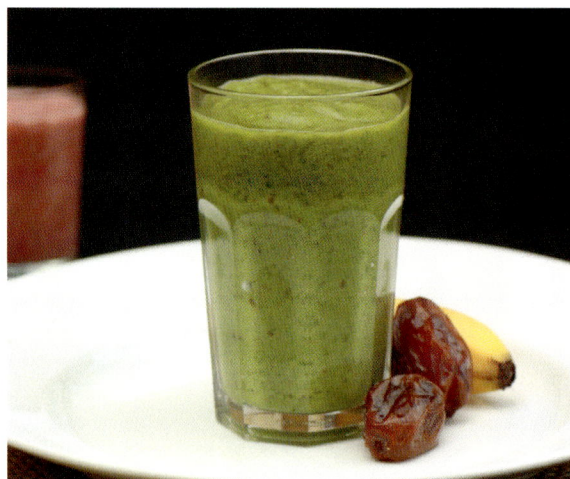

Kale? For breakfast? Yes indeed, and it's really tasty - even my 2-year-old loves this for a weekend breakfast treat! I prefer to use the milder green curly leaf variety of kale (versus the bumpy dinosaur "lacinato" or red varieties), or you can substitute spinach if kale is too bitter for your taste.

Serves 1

> 1/2 cup almond milk
> 1/4 cup water
> 1/4 large avocado, peeled
> 1-1/2 cups chopped fresh kale or spinach leaves
> 1/2 banana, peeled or 1/2 pear or apple, cored and quartered
> 1/2 cup ice cubes, crushed
> 2 dates, pitted or 2 Tablespoons maple syrup

1. Put all seven ingredients into a blender.
2. Blend for one minute, or until desired consistency is reached.
3. Pour into a tall glass and top with extra chopped dates if desired.

Turkey Apple Breakfast Sausage

Ground turkey, in my humble opinion, is totally underutilized by us amateur home chefs. If you're short on time in the mornings (and who isn't?), these savory little patties can be prepped the night before and cooked quickly the next morning for a hearty, warm breakfast.

Serves 2

> 1/2 pound ground turkey
> 1/2 cup shredded apple
> 2 Tablespoons rice cracker crumbs
> 1 Tablespoon sage leaf, crushed
> Dash of salt and pepper
> Dash of ground nutmeg
> Spoonful of mustard (optional)

1. In a large bowl combine the first six ingredients. Shape mixture into four 1/2-inch thick patties.
2. Arrange patties on lightly oiled pan. Broil 4-5 inches from the heat, about 10 minutes, or until no pink remains, turning once. (Or, heat olive oil in a skillet over medium heat and cook sausages for 8-10 minutes or until no pink remains.)
3. Remove from pan and serve with mustard on the side.

Tip: Make your own rice cracker crumbs by pulsing several rice crackers in the blender. They can often replace traditional bread crumbs in some of your favorite recipes.

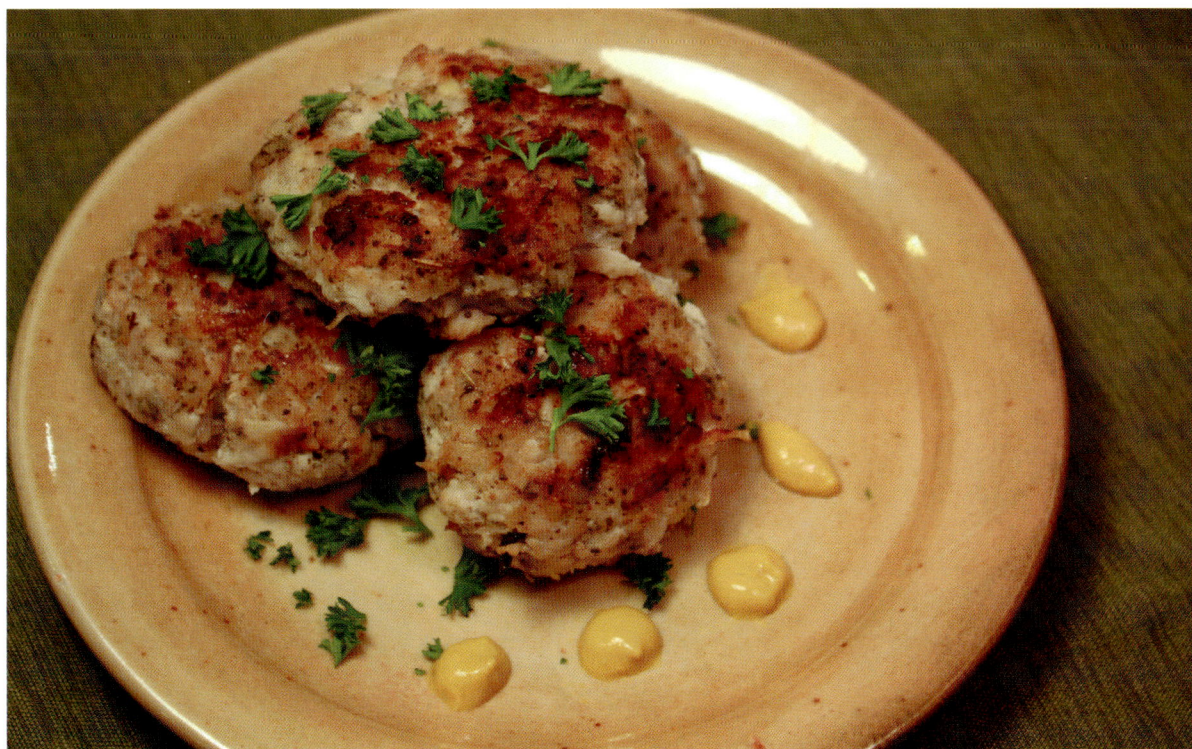

Pumpkin Pie Quinoa Bake

I don't normally enjoy sweet food first thing in the morning, but I'll always make an exception for this outstanding breakfast dish. Not only is it scrumptious, but it's also loaded with fiber and protein - talk about a power breakfast! It's quick to throw together so I like to bake this the night before while I'm cleaning up the dinner dishes, and then just reheat it in the morning. Inspired by www.healthfulpursuit.com

Serves 2

For the bake:

>   2/3 cup almond or rice milk
>   1/4 cup pumpkin puree or mashed sweet
>   potatoes
>   1/4 cup quinoa (yellow or red, or a mix of
>   both)
>   2 Tablespoons chopped dates (optional)
>   2 Tablespoons maple syrup
>   1 teaspoon coconut oil
>   1/4 teaspoon pure vanilla extract
>   1 teaspoon pumpkin pie spice

For the topping:

>   1 Tablespoon coconut oil, melted
>   2 Tablespoons maple syrup
>   2 Tablespoons finely ground almond flour
>   1/4 cup pecans or walnuts, chopped

1. Preheat oven to 350 degrees and lightly oil a small casserole dish or 2 large ramekins.
2. In a small bowl combine all the bake ingredients. Stir until fully mixed, then pour into the casserole dish or ramekins.
3. Cover and cook for 30 minutes.
4. Meanwhile, combine all topping ingredients. After the 30 minutes are up, remove casserole from oven and sprinkle topping over top of the casserole.
5. Return to the oven and cook uncovered for another 10-15 minutes, or until golden.

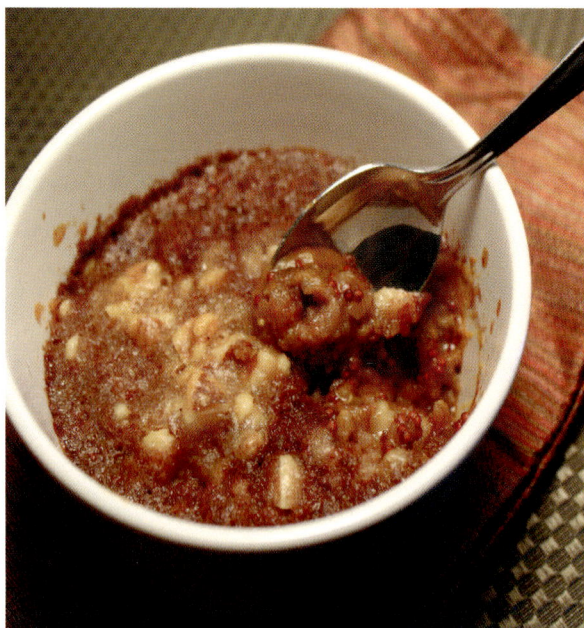

Millet, Rice & Quinoa Cereal

Nothing quite compares to a warm bowl of homemade cereal, and this is my favorite go-to recipe when I need a healthy start to the day. Add toppings based upon whatever is on hand in the pantry, and you'll find that it's fun to experiment with different combinations to find your own favorite. The leftover toasted grains from this recipe can be cooled and stored in a sealed container, so you can toast a big batch all at once to last the whole month. However, for the best nutrition, grind grains in a small electric coffee grinder or food processor just prior to cooking (they begin to lose nutritional value within 24-48 hours of grinding).

Inspired by Cynthia Lair

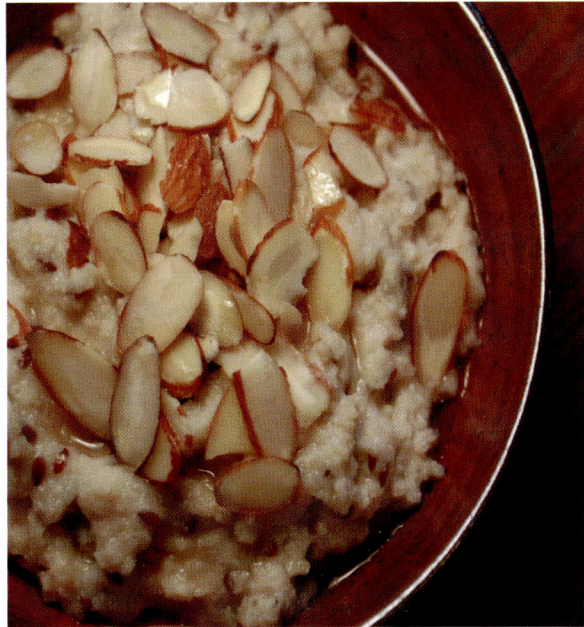

Serves 2

- 1 cup brown rice
- 1 cup millet
- 1 cup quinoa (yellow variety)
- 1 Tablespoon flax seeds
- 3 cups almond or rice milk, or water
- Optional toppings: more almond or rice milk, fruit, maple syrup, or nuts (almonds or walnuts)

1. Toast the rice, millet, and quinoa together: place grains in a large skillet and toast on medium heat, stirring the mixture constantly, until grains give off a nutty aroma (5-8 minutes).
2. Grind 2/3 cups of the mixture in a coffee grinder. In a pot, combine mixture, flax seeds, and the milk or water in a pot; bringing to a boil. Reduce heat to low and simmer, covered, for 10-12 minutes.
3. Top cereal with desired toppings and serve warm.

Fun Fact: Quinoa is a recently "rediscovered" ancient food native to South America where it was called the "gold of the Incas." They recognized its value in boosting the stamina of their warriors, but it's also appreciated nowadays as a unique "complete protein" grain.

Soups & Salads

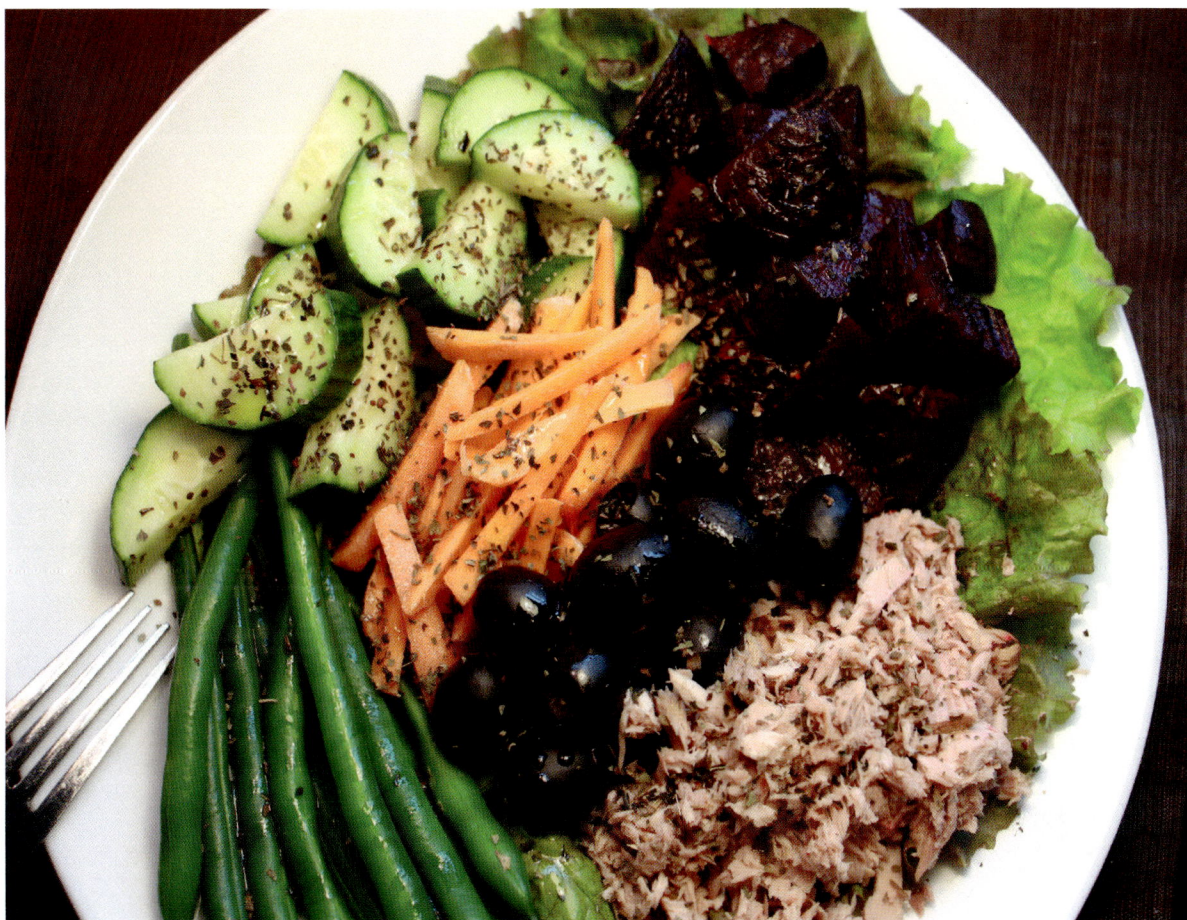

Salad Nicoise

Chinese Chicken Salad

Not much to say here except...yum! This is my favorite way to use up leftover plain chicken breasts, and watching my toddler pound the crackers to make crumbles is as much fun as eating this delicious salad!

Serves 4

2 chicken breasts, cooked and shredded
1 head nappa cabbage, thinly sliced and shredded
1 large carrot, grated
3 green onions, thinly sliced
1/2 cup toasted almonds, chopped
1/3 cup cilantro, chopped
2 Tablespoons toasted sesame seeds
15 brown rice crackers, crumbled

Dressing:
3 Tablespoons sesame oil
3 Tablespoons olive oil
1 to 2 Tablespoons brown rice syrup
2/3 cup rice vinegar
1/2 teaspoon salt
1/4 teaspoon pepper

1. Toss the first seven ingredients in a large bowl.
2. Mix the dressing ingredients in a small bowl and gently toss with the salad.
3. Sprinkle crackers over the salad.

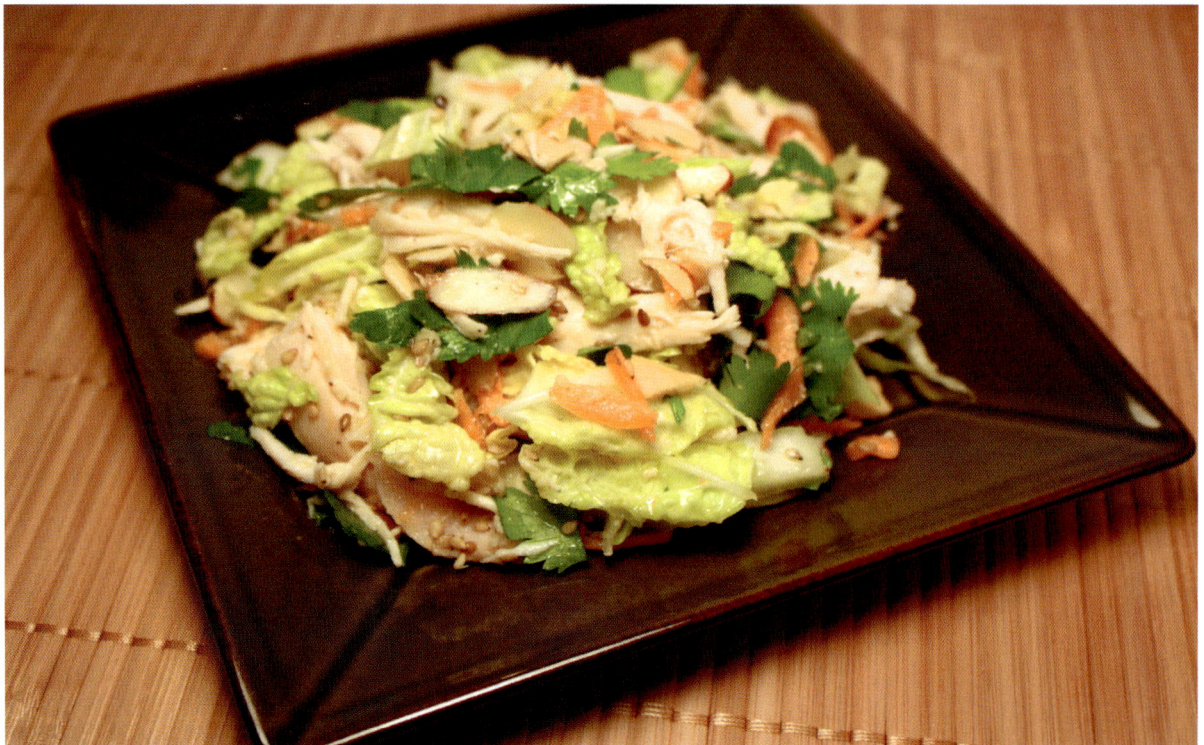

Salad Nicoise

There are as many variations of this French salad as there are cooks in France, I'm sure. This Elimination Diet-friendly version replaces the traditional eggs, potatoes, tomatoes and peppers with a fresh variety of vegetables that can be mixed and matched to suite both your own taste and what is in season at the market. Have fun composing this salad - I like concentric rows of the vegetables for a structured design, but freeform tossing looks great too!

Serves 4

- 1 head Romaine or Boston lettuce head, torn into bite-sized bits
- 2 beets, cooked and cubed (peeled optional)
- 1 cucumber, seeded and diced
- 1 large or 8 to 10 baby carrots, cut into thin strips
- 8 ounces cooked, cooled green beans
- 1 can black olives, drained
- 8 to 10-ounce can tuna packed in water, drained
- 1 large avocado, peeled, pitted, and diced
- 1/2 cup white beans (optional)
- Basil leaves to garnish (optional)

Vinaigrette dressing:
- 1 heaping Tablespoon spicy mustard
- 1 garlic clove, crushed
- 4 Tablespoons white wine vinegar
- 1/2 cup walnut oil or flax oil
- 1/4 to 1/2 cup olive oil
- Salt and pepper

1. Arrange the lettuce on a platter, top with the beets, cucumber, and carrots. Add green beans.
2. Arrange the olives, tuna, and avocado on top. Scatter white beans around the base and basil on top, if using.
3. Drizzle with vinaigrette and serve.

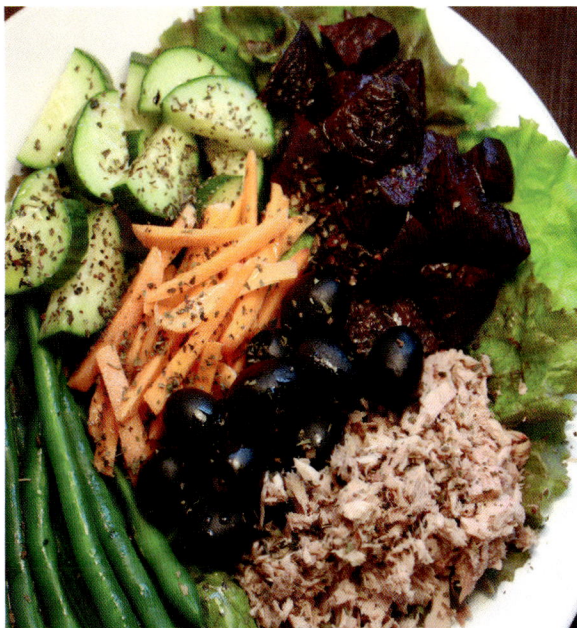

Southwestern Quinoa Salad

Can you say protein kick? Stuffed with protein-rich quinoa and beans, this salad makes for a hearty lunch or a nourishing post-workout meal. I love cumin and tend to lay it on heavy but if you have a more subtle palette then 1 tablespoon of the good stuff should satisfy your taste buds.

Serves 4

> 1-3/4 cups water or low-sodium chicken broth
> 1 cup quinoa
> 1 cup chickpeas (garbanzo beans)
> 1 cup cooked or canned black beans
> 1/2 cup diced red onion
> 2 cloves garlic, finely minced
> 1/2 cup cilantro, chopped
> 2 Tablespoons olive oil
> 1-2 Tablespoons cumin

1. Bring the water or stock to a boil in a medium saucepan over high heat. Add the quinoa and return to a boil. Reduce the heat to low, cover, and simmer for 20 minutes, or until quinoa is tender and the liquid is absorbed.
2. Meanwhile, in a large bowl, combine the remaining ingredients.
3. Add the quinoa and toss to coat well.

Tip: The simple addition of lime flavor renders this dish impossible to take just one bite of. For non-Elimination Dieters, add 1/4 cup lime juice to this salad when mixing and you'll see what I mean! The same thing goes for fresh diced tomatoes!

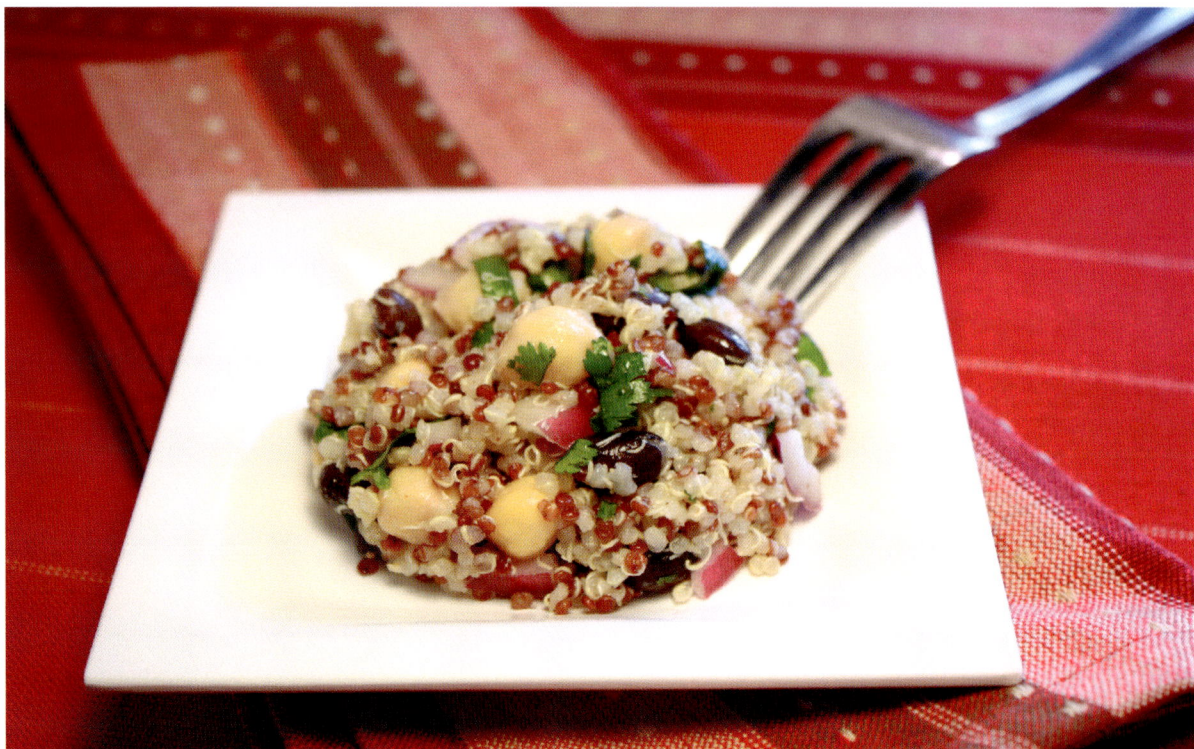

Strawberry Spinach Salad

Summer on a plate! Spinach and strawberries just seem to go hand in hand, both flavor and color. To elevate this salad to a main dish, just add shredded or chopped leftover chicken.

Serves 4

8 cups torn fresh spinach
1 pint fresh strawberries, sliced
1 cup thinly sliced cucumber
1/4 cup red onion, julienned
1/4 cup slivered almonds

Dressing:
1/2 cup olive oil
3 Tablespoons honey or brown rice syrup
1/4 cup apple cider vinegar or champagne vinegar
1 Tablespoon poppy seeds
1/4 teaspoon pepper
1-1/2 teaspoons finely chopped onion or shallot

1. Divide spinach, strawberries, cucumber, and red onion between four plates.
2. Combine dressing ingredients in a small bowl. Blend, then dress the salads.
3. Top with slivered almonds.

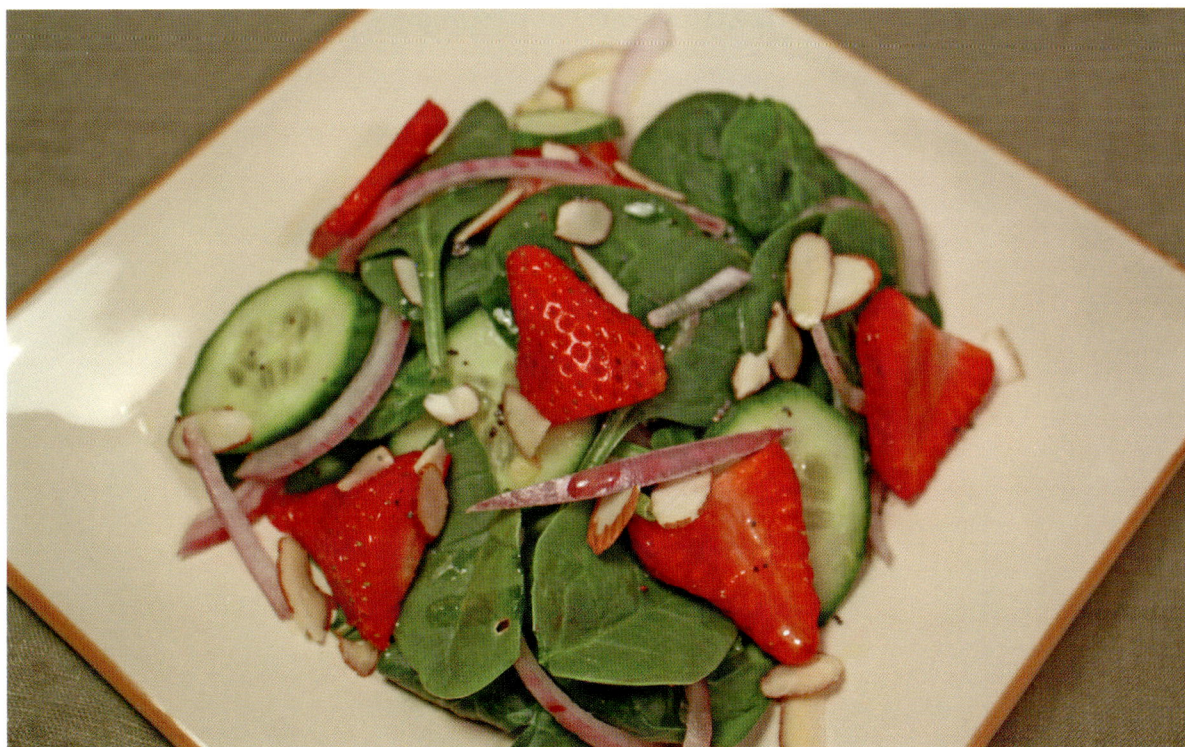

Pear Harvest Salad

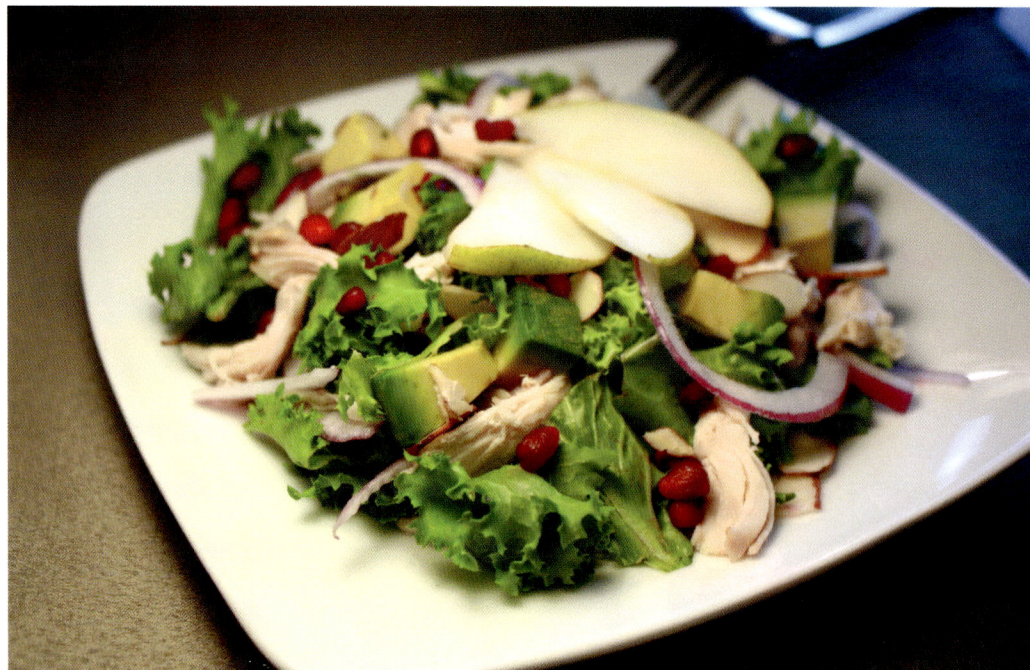

Your quest for the perfect Thanksgiving leftovers meal is over - this salad makes the most of holiday favorites like turkey, pears, and pomegranates. It's so good that I buy a bird a few pounds larger than the number of folks I'm serving just to ensure that I'll have plenty of meat left to enjoy this perfect holiday hangover cure.

Serves 6

> 2 packages (5-ounces each) spring mix salad greens
> 4 cups cubed or shredded cooked turkey breast
> 2 medium pears, sliced
> 1 medium ripe avocado, peeled and cubed
> 1/2 cup pomegranate seeds
> 1/2 small red onion, thinly sliced
> 1/2 cup sliced almonds, roasted

> Dressing:
> 1/2 cup olive oil
> 3 Tablespoons honey or brown rice syrup
> 1 Tablespoon red wine vinegar
> 1 Tablespoon spicy mustard
> 1/2 teaspoon salt
> 1/2 teaspoon pepper

1. Divide spring mix among six plates.
2. Top with turkey pears, avocado, pomegranate seeds and onion.
3. Whisk the dressing ingredients; drizzle over salads. Sprinkle with almonds and serve.

Tip: For non-Elimination Dieters, a few crumbles of blue cheese or goat cheese are a very welcome addition to this salad.

Chicken & Pasta Broth

This homemade version of chicken noodle soup is guaranteed to please! My family often requests this on snowy winter evenings or when recovering from a head cold - the very essence of "comfort food," no?

Serves 6

- 12 ounces boneless chicken breasts
- 2 Tablespoons olive oil
- 1 medium onion, diced
- 1-1/2 cups carrots, diced
- 9 ounces cauliflower florets (about 4 cups)
- 3-1/4 cups chicken stock
- 3 teaspoons dried mixed herbs or 3 Tablespoons chopped fresh mixed herbs
- 1-1/4 cups small rice pasta shapes
- Salt and pepper
- Parsley for garnish

1. Finely dice the chicken breasts with a sharp knife. Remove and discard any skin.
2. Heat the oil in a large heavy bottomed pan or skillet over a medium-high heat. Add the diced chicken and the onion, carrots, and cauliflower. Sauté until they are lightly colored.
3. Stir in the chicken stock and herbs. Bring to a boil and add the pasta shapes. Return to boil. Cover, and simmer for 10 minutes, stirring occasionally to prevent the pasta shapes sticking together.
4. Season to taste with salt and pepper, garnish with parsley.

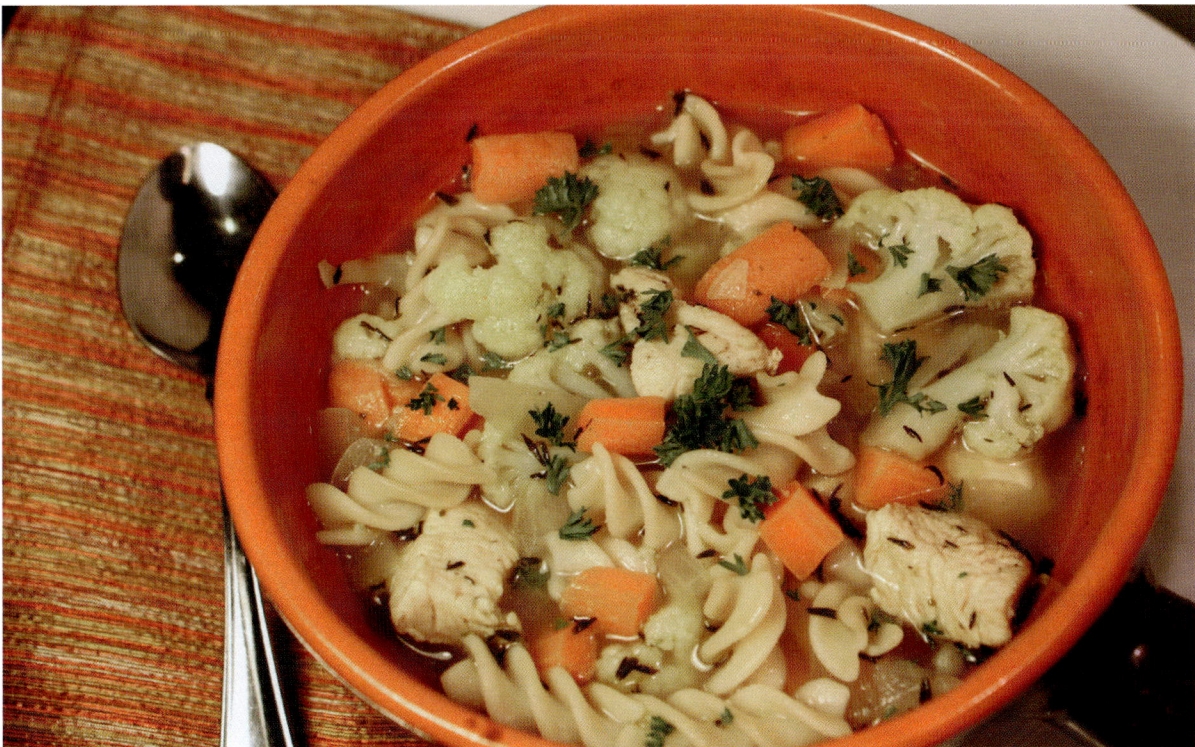

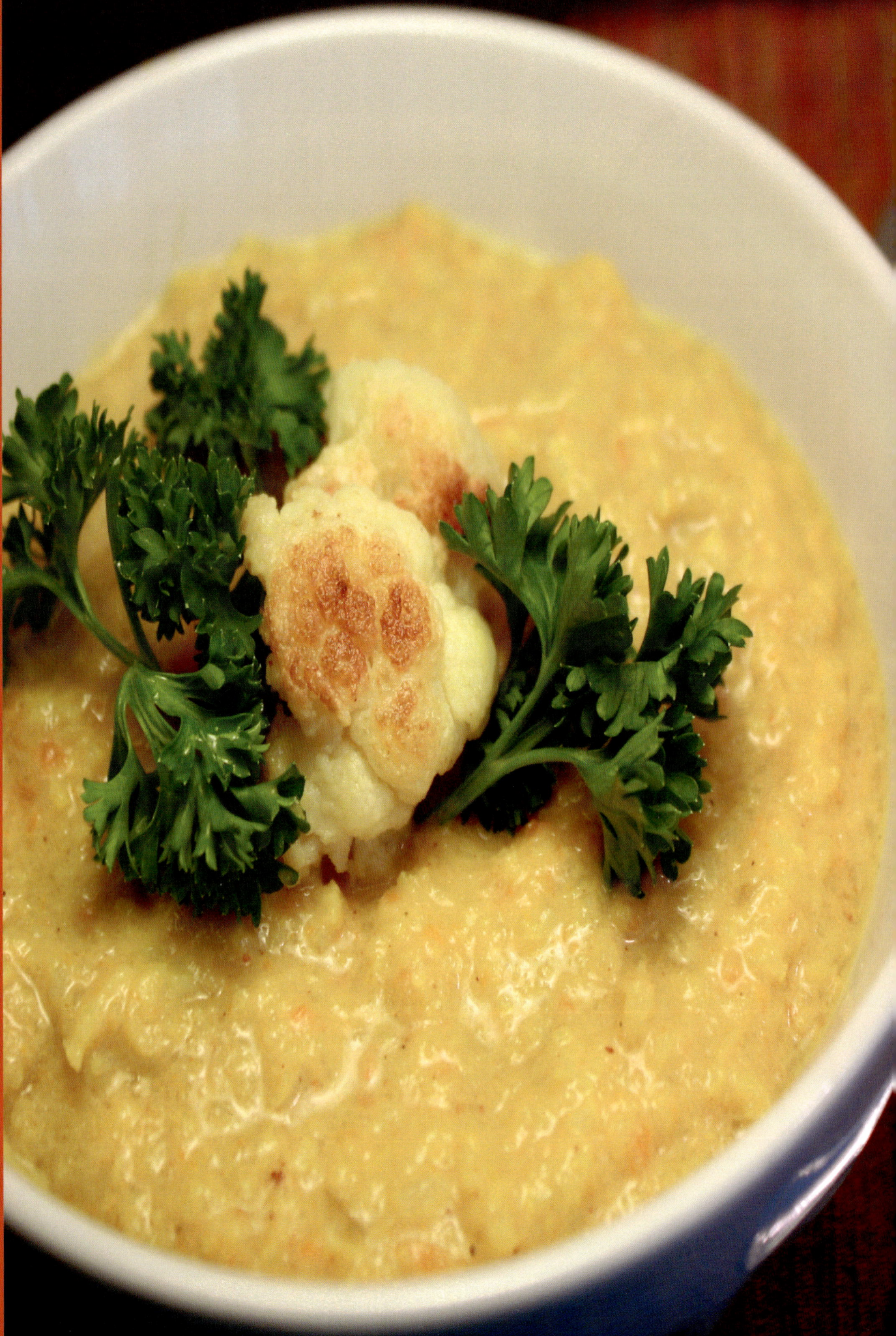

Curried Vegetable Soup

This hearty soup was inspired by my husband's co-worker, Erin, who also provided all the wonderful photos in this book! She's always sending me lovely recipes to trial and swap ideas about, and this is an adaptation of one of her delicious recipes.

Adapted from Erin Seyfried

Serves 4

1 head cauliflower, cut into florets and the stem into chunks
2 carrots (or 12-16 baby carrots), chunked into similar size as cauliflower florets
5 Tablespoons olive oil, divided
Salt and pepper
1 medium onion, chopped
4 garlic cloves, crushed
1 Tablespoon curry powder
1 teaspoon ground ginger
1 teaspoon ground cumin
2 Tablespoons flour (almond, rice, or quinoa)
1 cup almond, rice, or light coconut milk
4 cups low-sodium chicken or vegetable broth
1 cup shredded chicken (optional)
1 cup frozen peas, thawed (optional)
Cilantro, to garnish

1. Preheat oven to 425 degrees. Toss cauliflower and carrots with 1 tablespoon olive oil, salt and pepper. Roast on an aluminum-foil lined baking sheet for 20 minutes until tender and golden, turning after ten minutes.
2. In a large stock pot, heat 1 tablespoon olive oil over medium heat. Add the onion and cook for 5 minutes, until softened. Add the garlic, curry powder, ginger, and cumin. Cook, stirring constantly for 1-2 minutes more, being careful not to burn the garlic. Remove mixture to a small bowl.
3. In the same pot, heat 3 tablespoons olive oil over medium-low heat. Add the flour gradually and blend well to form a paste. Once slightly bubbling, add the milk gradually (about 1/2 cup at a time) and blend or whisk to eliminate clumps. Once the mixture begins to thicken, gradually add the chicken broth. Bring mixture to a simmer.
4. Add the onion and cauliflower mixtures from the first two steps to the soup, reserving a few florets to garnish, simmer for 10 minutes. Using an immersion blender or food processor, puree soup to desired consistency. Return to pot and add chicken and peas, if using.
5. Serve, with reserved cauliflower florets and cilantro as garnish.

Tip: For this recipe any non-dairy milk will do, but coconut milk and curry are natural partners. You can purchase light coconut milk in the grocery store, but it's cheaper to purchase regular coconut milk and just dilute it yourself with water (which is all that canned light coconut milk really is) - the remaining canned coconut milk can be frozen and thawed later for future use.

Butternut Squash Soup

The soup that started it all! This was my very first published recipe (in the October/ November 2009 Taste of Home *magazine), and the mere act of being published really boosted my confidence to create this cookbook. I hope you enjoy this rich, comforting soup as much as my family does!*

Serves 6

One 3-1/2 pound butternut squash peeled, seeded, and cut into 1-inch cubes
2 teaspoons salt
1/2 teaspoon ground black pepper
3 Tablespoons olive oil, divided
1 Tablespoon olive oil

2 cups onion, chopped
2 cups celery, chopped
1/4 to 1/3 cup chopped fresh sage, or 2 to 3 Tablespoon dried sage
6 cups chicken broth
24 fresh, large whole sage leaves
Olive oil to fry

1. Preheat oven to 400 degrees. In a large bowl, toss the squash with salt, pepper, and 2 tablespoons of olive oil.
2. Place the squash on a rimmed baking sheet and roast in oven for 15 minutes. Stir the cubes and continue roasting for 15 minutes or until they are caramelized and easily pricked with a fork; then set aside.
3. In a Dutch oven or a large stockpot, heat the remaining 1 tablespoon olive oil over medium heat. Add the onion, celery, and sage and sauté, stirring occasionally, until the vegetables are translucent and tender, 10 minutes. Add the squash and broth and bring to a boil. Lower heat and simmer for 30 minutes or until the liquid is flavorful. Remove from heat.
4. Using a blender or a food processor, blend the soup in batches until smooth. Return to the pot and keep warm.
5. To make fried sage leaves, heat olive oil on medium high. When the oil is hot, add several of the sage leaves and fry in batches. When slightly crispy, remove from oil with tongs and drain on a paper towel.
6. Dish out soup in bowls and garnish with 4 sage leaves each.

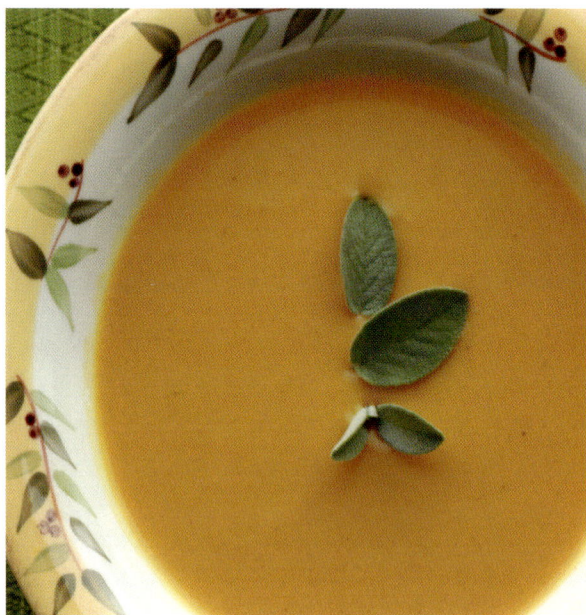

Black Bean Brew

Dried beans are a great choice for the economical home cook, averaging only half to two-thirds of the price of canned beans. If you can plan ahead to cook dried beans, just prepare a large batch and freeze whatever you don't need for the recipe - they'll keep just fine in the freezer for a few months.

Adapted from *www.bettycrocker.com*

Serves 6

1 cup dry black beans
8 cups water, divided
2 cups chicken broth
1 cup chopped onion (1 large)
1 cup chopped celery (3 stalks)
4 cloves garlic, minced
2 teaspoons ground cumin
1/4 teaspoon salt
1/4 teaspoon pepper
8 ounces cooked chicken, shredded
1 large avocado, diced
Snipped fresh cilantro

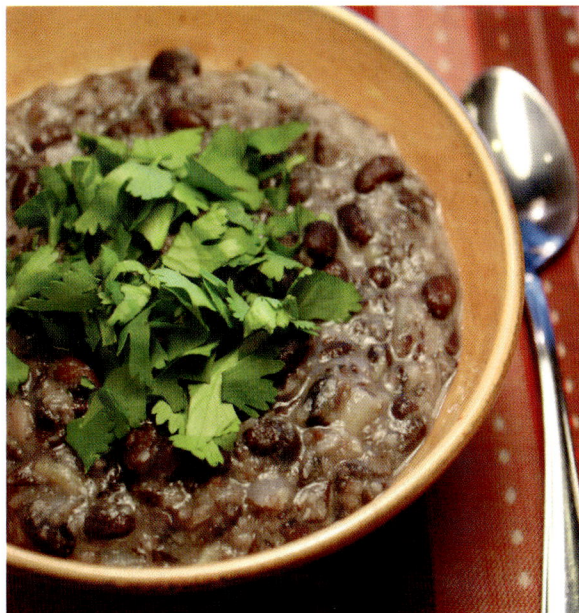

1. Rinse beans. In a large saucepan or pot combine beans and 6 cups water. Bring to boil, reduce heat. Simmer for 2 minutes. Remove from heat. Cover and let stand for 1 hour. (Or, place beans in water in pan. Cover and let soak in a cool place for 6 to 8 hours or overnight.) Drain and rinse beans.
2. In the same pan combine beans, chicken broth, remaining 2 cups water, onion, celery, garlic, cumin, salt, and pepper. Bring to boiling; reduce heat. Cover and simmer for 1 hour or until beans are tender.
3. Mash beans slightly, if desired. Stir in chicken and avocado. Cook 2-3 minutes more or until heated through. Garnish with fresh cilantro.

Tip: If you're in a rush, try the "shortcut" version: Prepare as above, except omit dry black beans and the 6 cups soaking water, decrease chicken broth to 1-1/2 cups. Rinse and drain two 15-ounce cans of black beans, add to saucepan with broth, the 2 cups water, vegetables, and seasonings. Bring to boil; reduce heat. Cover and simmer about 15 minutes or till vegetables are tender. Finish with step 3 above.

Cauliflower Bisque

Paired with a small salad, this rich and creamy soup is wonderful for a simple weeknight meal. It also freezes well for those inevitable evenings when defrosting in the microwave is the most work you're willing to exert in the kitchen. Sunset Magazine describes the cauliflower flavor as very mild, and it's true - even if you don't normally enjoy cauliflower, you will surely enjoy this!

Adapted from www.sunset.com

Serves 4-6

3 Tablespoons olive oil, divided
2 medium onions, halved and thinly sliced
1/2 teaspoon salt
3 garlic cloves, minced
4-1/2 cups chicken or vegetable broth, divided
1 large head cauliflower (2 pounds), chopped
Ground white pepper
2 Tablespoons minced chives
1 Tablespoon finely chopped flat-leaf parsley

1. Heat 1 tablespoon olive oil in a large pot over medium-high heat. Add onions and salt, cover, reduce heat to medium, and cook, stirring occasionally, until onions are very soft, 5 to 8 minutes. Add garlic and 1/2 cup chicken broth. Cook, stirring, until liquid is almost completely evaporated, 3 to 5 minutes.
2. Stir in cauliflower and remaining 4 cups broth and bring to a boil. Reduce heat to a simmer, cover, and cook until cauliflower is very soft, 20-25 minutes.
3. Using a blender, mix soup until smooth. (Or, if you like it chunky, pulse to blend). Season to taste with white pepper and salt. Ladle soup into bowls.
4. In a small bowl, combine the remaining 2 tablespoons olive oil, chives, and parsley. Drizzle on top of soup.

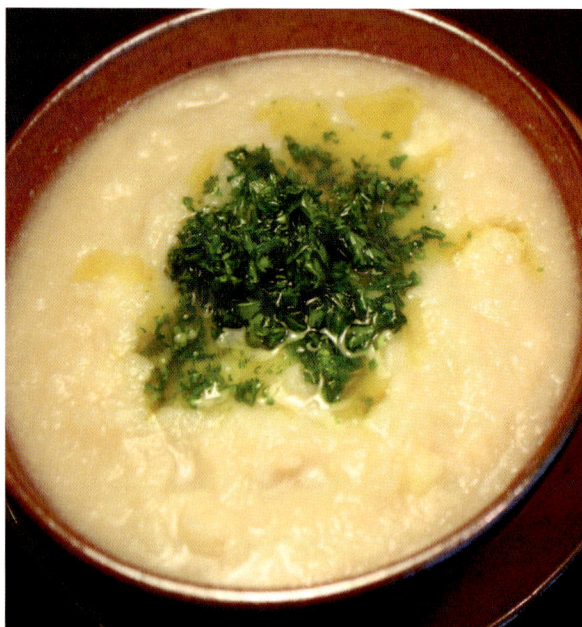

Poultry & Meats

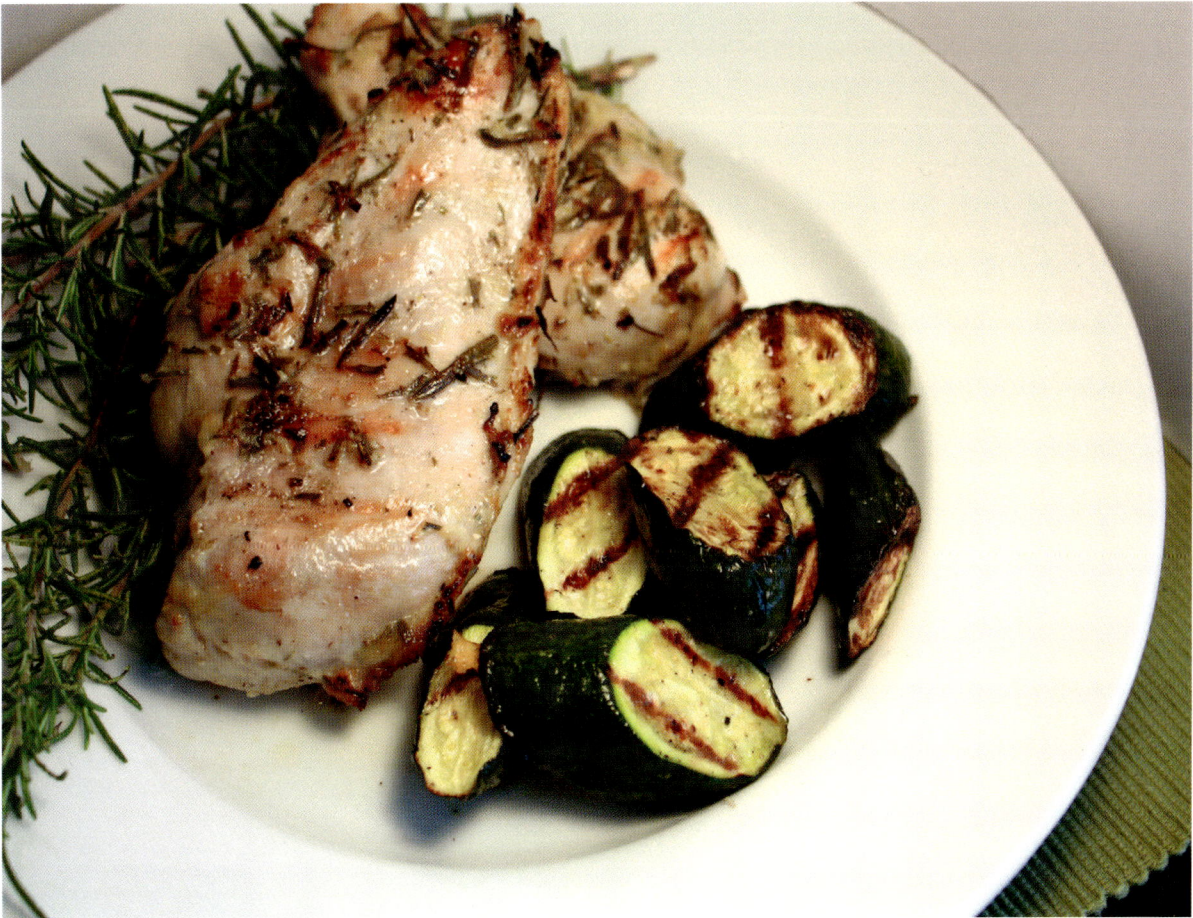

Tuscan BBQ Chicken

Smothered Chicken

This simple meal makes use of basic kitchen staples but somehow tastes extra special. It also reheats well and makes wonderful leftovers, so feel free to double-up on the ingredients and enjoy an easy mid-week lunch the next day!

Serves 4

- 4 cups fresh baby spinach
- 2 cups sliced fresh mushrooms
- 3 green onions, sliced
- 3 Tablespoons chopped pecans, toasted
- 2 teaspoon olive oil
- 4 boneless chicken breast halves (4 ounces each)
- 2 teaspoons herbes de Provence

1. In a large skillet, sauté the spinach, mushrooms, green onions, and pecans in olive oil until mushrooms are tender. Set aside and keep warm.
2. Sprinkle chicken with herbes de Provence. Grill chicken, covered, over medium heat or broil 4 inches from the heat for 6-8 minutes on each side.
3. To serve, top each chicken breast with reserved spinach mixture.

Tip: For non-Elimination Dieters, you can add a thin slice of provolone or mozzarella cheese on top of the grilled chicken before smothering with the spinach mixture (then cover to let cheese melt). The cheese mixes beautifully with the spinach mixture and creates a truly luxurious dish!

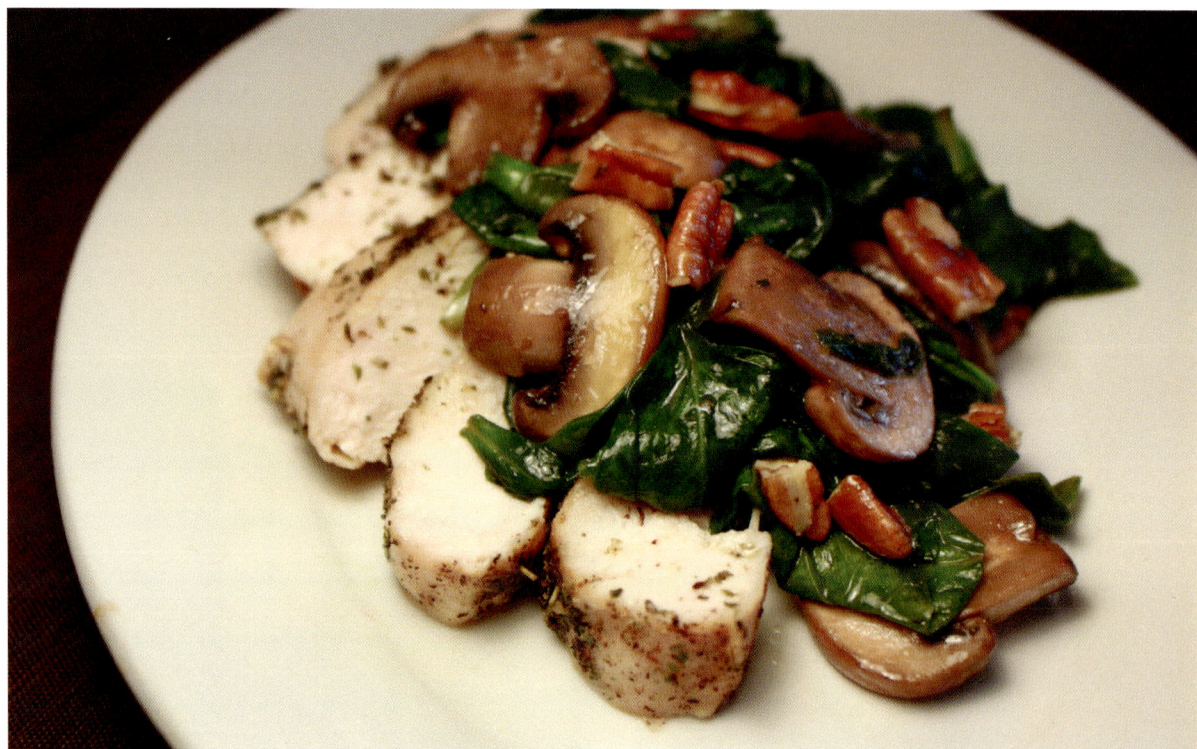

Chicken Packets

Everyone has a go-to recipe for company, and this is mine. It never fails to impress guests with its unusual presentation and it always comes out of the oven perfectly cooked. The best part? The packets can be prepared a day in advance and then cooked while you're serving appetizers and visiting with your guests. Make sure to place the ingredients on the shiny side of the foil (so that the dull side faces out when the packet is wrapped up) to ensure that the heat is absorbed into the parcel and not reflected away.

Serves 4

> Olive oil
> 4 skinless chicken breasts
> 4 small zucchini, sliced vertically into
>   1/2 inch slices, divided
> Pepper
> 1 small bunch fresh basil or dried basil,
>   divided
> 12-16 large mushrooms, thinly sliced
> Rice or rice pasta to serve (optional)

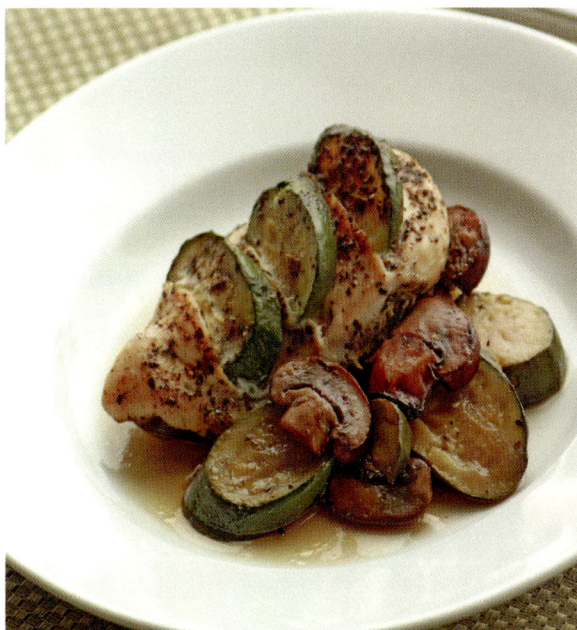

1. Preheat oven to 400 degrees.
2. Cut 6 pieces of foil, each measuring about 10 inches square. Lightly drizzle the center of the foil squares lightly with oil and set aside.
3. With a sharp knife, slash each chicken breast at 3 regular intervals. Place one zucchini slice between the each cut in the chicken. Sprinkle with pepper and basil.
4. Divide the remaining zucchini and mushrooms between the pieces of foil and sprinkle with pepper to taste. Tear or roughly chop the basil and scatter over the vegetables in each parcel.
5. Place the chicken on top of each pile of vegetables, then wrap in the foil to enclose the chicken and vegetables, tucking in the ends.
6. Place on a cookie sheet and bake for about 30-45 minutes.
7. To serve, unwrap each foil parcel and, if desired, serve with rice or rice pasta to soak up the juices.

Tip: For non-Elimination Dieters, try replacing the zucchini slices inserted into the chicken in Step 3 with thin slices of mozzarella cheese. Yum!

Turkey Cutlets with Blackberry Sauce

This is a fantastic weeknight supper, as both the turkey and sauce can be prepared at the same time in less than 10 minutes. I usually make a double-batch of the sauce, as it freezes very well and can be used to top a wide range of meats. Chinese five-spice powder is easy to find pre-packaged in the spice aisle or Asian food section of the grocery store or online, but if you're a DIY-er, a recipe for Chinese five-spice powder is listed below.

Serves 4

> 1 pound turkey or chicken cutlets
> Salt and pepper
> 2 Tablespoons apple cider vinegar
> 1-1/2 cups blackberries, fresh or frozen
> 1/4 teaspoon ground cinnamon
> 1/2 teaspoon Chinese five-spice powder
>   (see below)
> 1/8 teaspoon black pepper
> 1 to 2 Tablespoons honey or brown rice
>   syrup
> 1/4 cup olive oil

1. Sprinkle cutlets with salt and pepper to taste. Cook cutlets in an oiled grill or frying pan at medium heat for about 3-4 minutes per side, or until there are no traces of pink in the middle.
2. Meanwhile, place the next six ingredients in a blender and blend on high for several minutes. Turn blender to low and add olive oil in a gentle continuous stream and let it fully blend into the mixture.
3. Drizzle sauce over turkey cutlets to serve.

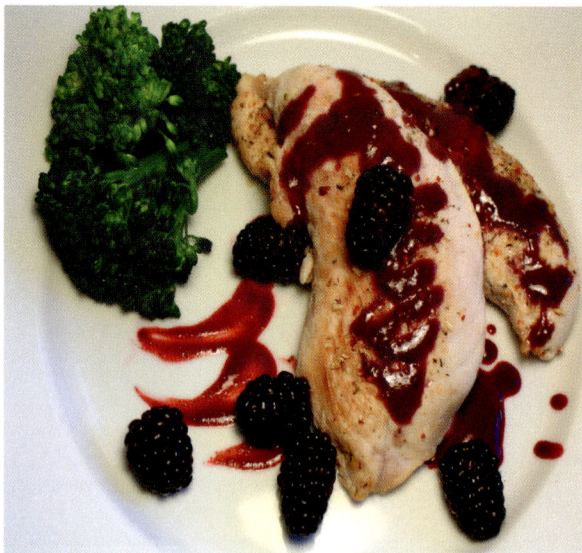

Chinese Five-Spice Powder recipe

> 1 teaspoon ground Szechwan pepper or regular black pepper
> 1 teaspoon ground star anise
> 1-1/4 teaspoon ground fennel seeds
> 1/2 teaspoon ground cloves
> 1/2 teaspoon ground cinnamon
> 1/2 teaspoon salt
> 1/4 teaspoon ground white pepper

1. Combine all ingredients and store in a cool, dark area.

Chicken Provence

This dish competes as one of my all-time forever favorites - it's scrumptious, embarrassingly easy to prepare, and makes for an impressive presentation. I often prep this the night before and throw it oven when I get home from work. 45 unattended minutes later...voila! If you haven't yet been introduced to leeks, prepare to be dazzled!

Adapted from *www.realsimple.com*

Serves 4

> 8 bone-in chicken thighs and breasts (about 2-1/2 to 3 pounds)
> 4 red apples, cored and quartered
> 3 to 4 large leeks (white/light green parts only),
>   rinsed, halved crosswise and length wise
> 8 sprigs fresh rosemary
> 2 Tablespoons olive oil
> 1/4 teaspoon salt
> 3/4 teaspoon pepper

1. Preheat oven to 400 degrees.
2. On a large rimmed baking sheet (or in a large roasting pan), toss all of the ingredients. Turn the chicken skin-side up.
3. Roast until the chicken is cooked through and the apples and leeks are tender, 40-45 minutes.

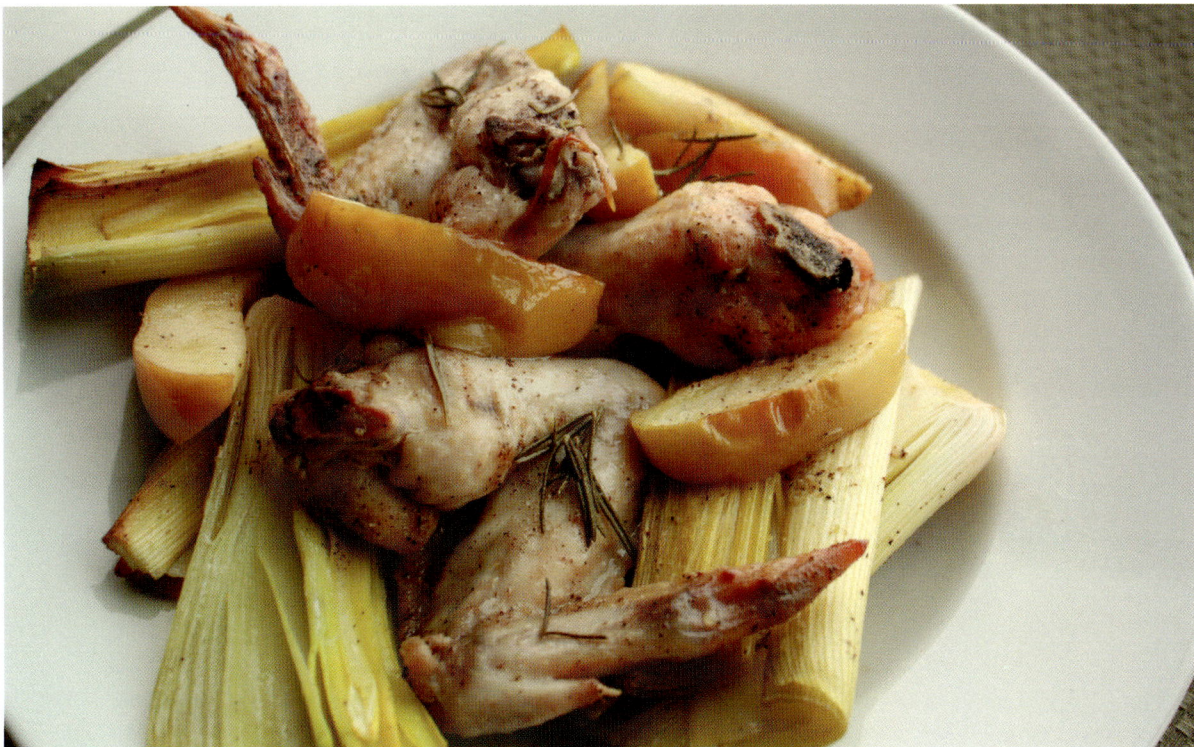

Roasted Cornish Game Hens

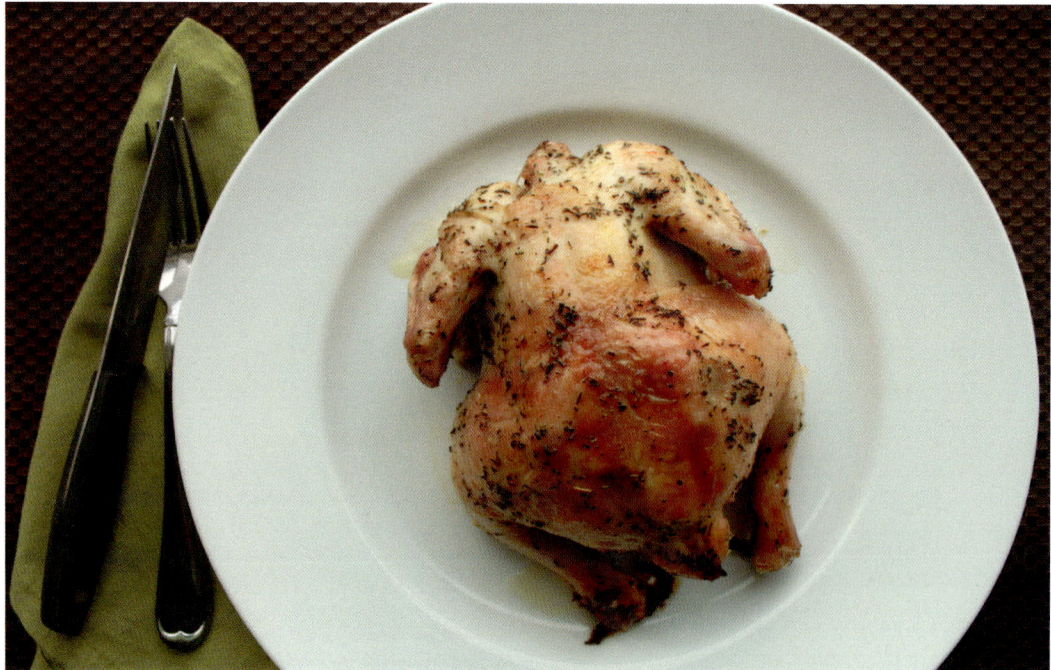

These little guys can seem intimidating to the uninitiated chef, but I assure you that they couldn't be easier to make nor impress your guests with - you'll never see dinner disappear so quickly! Be sure not to crowd the hens on the baking sheets so the skins crisp up properly and they take minimal time to cook through.

Serves 2

> 2 teaspoons salt
> 1 teaspoon pepper
> 1 teaspoon dried basil
> 1 teaspoon dried thyme
> 1 Tablespoon olive oil
> 2 Cornish game hens, 1-1/2 pounds each, livers and gizzards removed
> 1 small carrot, diced
> 1 stalk celery, chopped
> 1/2 onion or 2 shallots, diced
> 1 teaspoon dried thyme

1. Preheat oven to 375 degrees.
2. In a small mixing bowl, stir together salt, pepper, basil, and thyme. Rub olive oil all over the hens and season each with the salt mixture. Place the hens on a foil-lined baking sheet pan with space between each hen.
3. Combine the carrot, celery, onion, and thyme. Loosely stuff the cavities of each hen with some of the vegetable mixture.
4. Roast the hens in the preheated oven for about 1 hour or until the thickest part of the thigh registers 165 degrees and the juices run clear.
5. Remove the hens from the oven, loosely cover with foil and let rest 10 minutes before carving or serving.

Tuscan BBQ Chicken

Rosemary grows like a weed in many areas, so you can likely step out your front door and locate some quicker in your neighborhood than jumping in the car and heading to the grocery store! This dish makes for a convenient complete meal when grilled and served alongside some zucchini, squash, or eggplant (the veggies have a shorter grill time, though, so they should be thrown on the grill with the chicken once it's halfway cooked).

Adapted from *www.marthastewartliving.com*

Serves 4

1/2 cup water
1/4 cup chopped fresh rosemary or 2 Tablespoons dried rosemary
1/4 cup olive oil
4 cloves garlic
Salt and pepper
4 large chicken breasts or 12 chicken thighs.

1. In a small saucepan, bring the water and rosemary to a boil; remove from heat, cover, and let steep 5 minutes. Transfer to a blender. Add oil and garlic; season with salt and pepper. Puree into a marinade until smooth; let cool.
2. Combine chicken and rosemary marinade in a shallow dish and turn to coat. Cover, and let it marinate at least 15 minutes at room temperature or overnight in the refrigerator, turning chicken occasionally.
3. Remove chicken from marinade and place on grill or grill pan. Discard marinade. Cook chicken, turning as needed to prevent burning, until cooked throughout, about 20 minutes.

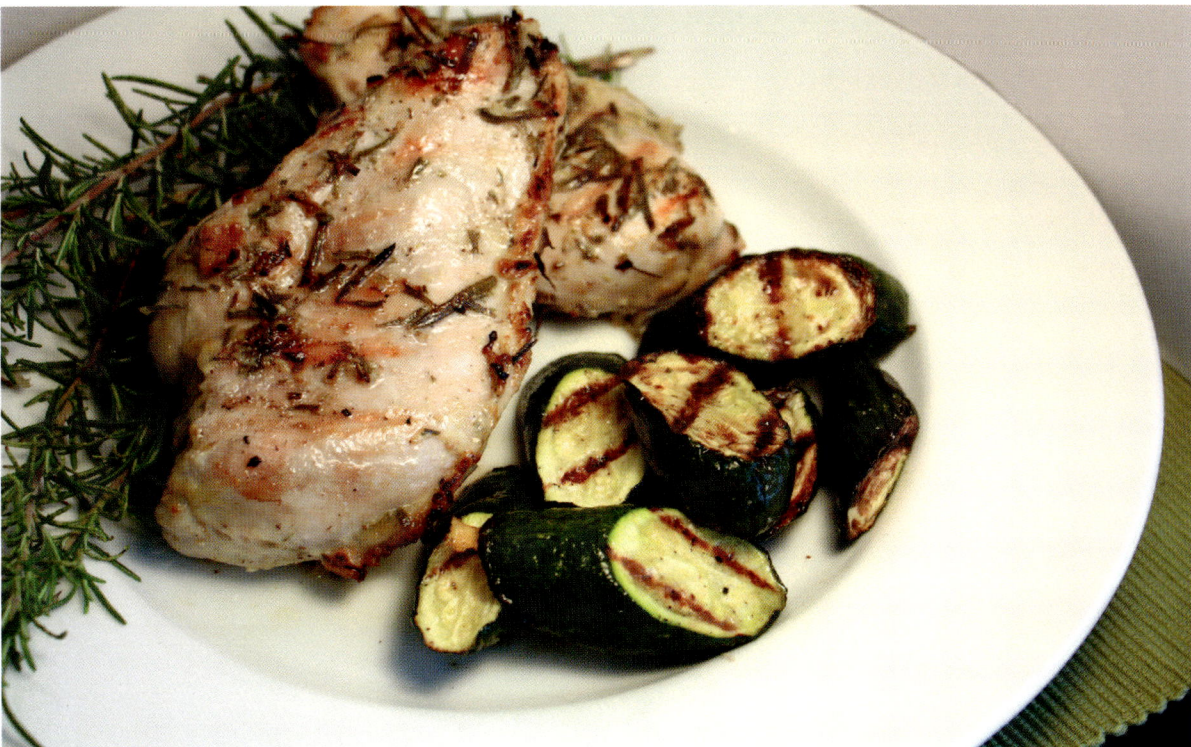

Turkey Burgers with Cranberry Sauce

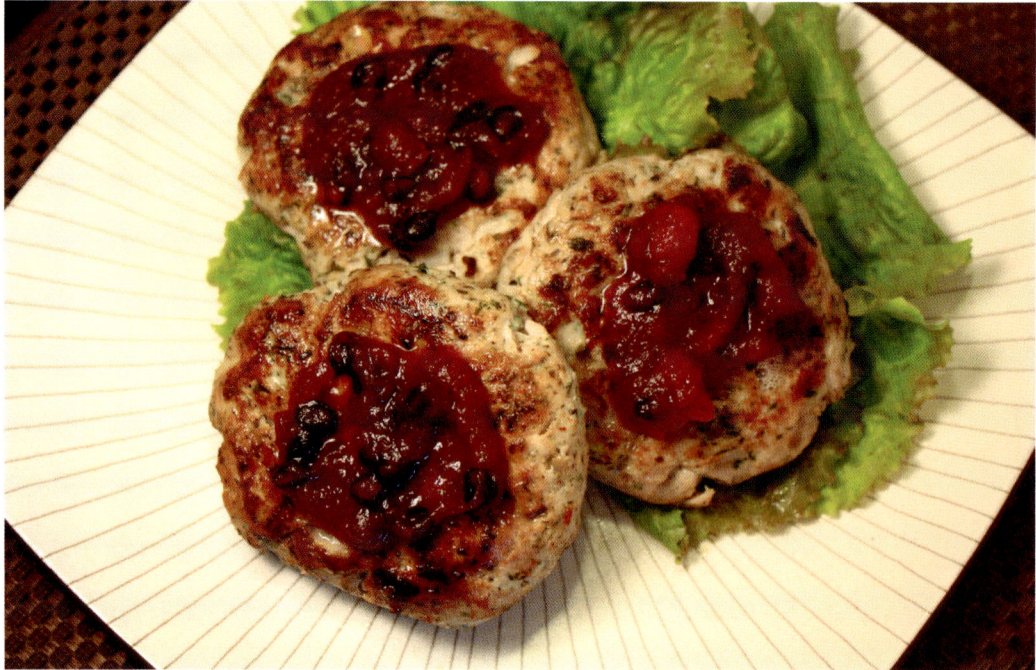

No need to wait for Thanksgiving to enjoy delicious and anti-oxidant-packed cranberries! This simple recipe can be made year-round thanks to frozen cranberries in the grocery store's frozen foods aisle. I like to add a pinch of cinnamon or cloves to my sauce, but the basic recipe is wonderful as-is to accompany these savory patties.

Serves 4

- 1-1/4 pounds ground turkey
- 1 small onion or 2 shallots, chopped (1/2 cup)
- 1 Tablespoon spicy mustard
- 2 Tablespoons each parsley, sage, and thyme, chopped (or 2 teaspoon each dried)
- 1 teaspoon salt
- 1/2 teaspoon pepper
- 1 Tablespoon olive oil
- One 12-ounce bag cranberries (2 cups frozen)
- 1 cup water
- 1/2 cup honey or brown rice syrup
- 1/4 cup pomegranate seeds (optional)

1. Make the burgers: in a large bowl, combine first six ingredients. Shape into four patties.
2. Heat olive oil in a large skillet over medium-high heat and cook patties for 5-6 minutes on each side.
3. Meanwhile, make the sauce: combine cranberries, water, honey, and pomegranates (if using) in a sauce pan. Bring to a boil, reduce temperature to simmer for 5-6 minutes until cranberries pop and the sauce thickens.
4. Serve sauce over grilled patties.

Chicken Sausage Patties

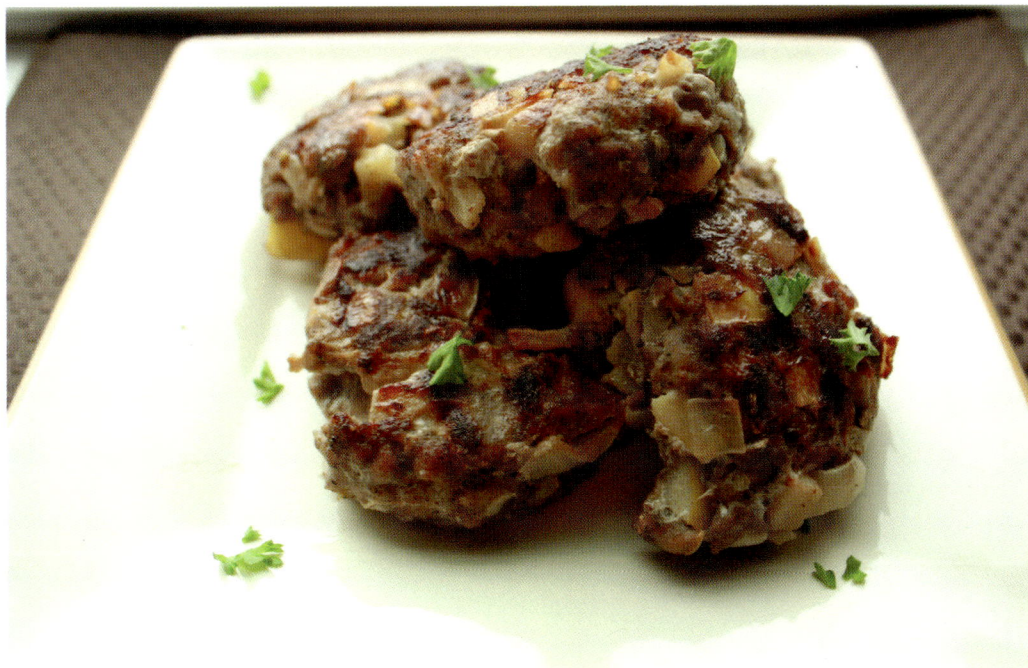

I was always a bit baffled by ground chicken in the meat aisle, until I tried this recipe! Prepared and seasoned correctly, ground chicken makes an excellent alternative to ground beef hamburgers. These little patties are the proof!

Serves 4 (3 patties each)

> 1 Tablespoon olive oil
> 1 green apple, finely chopped
> 1 small onion, finely chopped
> Salt and pepper, to taste
> 1 teaspoon fennel seed
> 1-1/2 pounds ground chicken breast
> 1-1/2 teaspoons poultry seasoning
> 1 teaspoon allspice
> 1 teaspoon garlic powder (optional
> Olive oil, for drizzling

1. Heat a small nonstick skillet over medium heat. Add olive oil. Add apple and onion and season with salt, pepper and fennel seeds. Gently sauté the mixture 5 minutes to soften and remove from heat to cool.
2. Heat a grill pan or large nonstick skillet over medium-high heat.
3. Place chicken in a bowl and season with salt and pepper, poultry seasoning, allspice, garlic powder (if using) and a long drizzle of olive oil. Add in the apples, onions and fennel and mix well with hands.
4. Divide meat into 4 sections and form 3 small, thin patties from each section (12 patties total).
5. Cook patties 3-4 minutes on each side and serve warm.

Roasted Leg of Lamb

Looking to prepare a classic but low-stress Sunday or holiday brunch? This dish relies on basic pantry staples (except for the lamb itself!) and easy preparation, so it's pretty hard to mess up. Lamb is traditionally served in spring, but a good butcher should be able to locate an excellent cut for you any time of the year.

Serves 6

> **One leg of lamb (4 to 6 pounds)**
> **3 cloves garlic, peeled and slivered**
> **1/3 cup olive oil**
> **1/3 cup spicy mustard**
> **2 teaspoon salt**
> **3 Tablespoons dried rosemary**
> **Pepper**
> **2 to 4 sprigs fresh rosemary**

1. Preheat oven to 425 degrees.
2. Using a paring knife, make small incisions in the skin of the lamb. Insert the garlic slivers in the slits.
3. Mix the olive oil and mustard and rub it over the entire leg of lamb. Sprinkle with the salt, rosemary, and pepper.
4. Roast the lamb for 45-55 minutes or until internal temperature reaches 135 degrees. Remove from the oven, cover with foil and let rest for 20 minutes. Carve the lamb in thin slices and serve with pan juices and fresh rosemary sprigs.

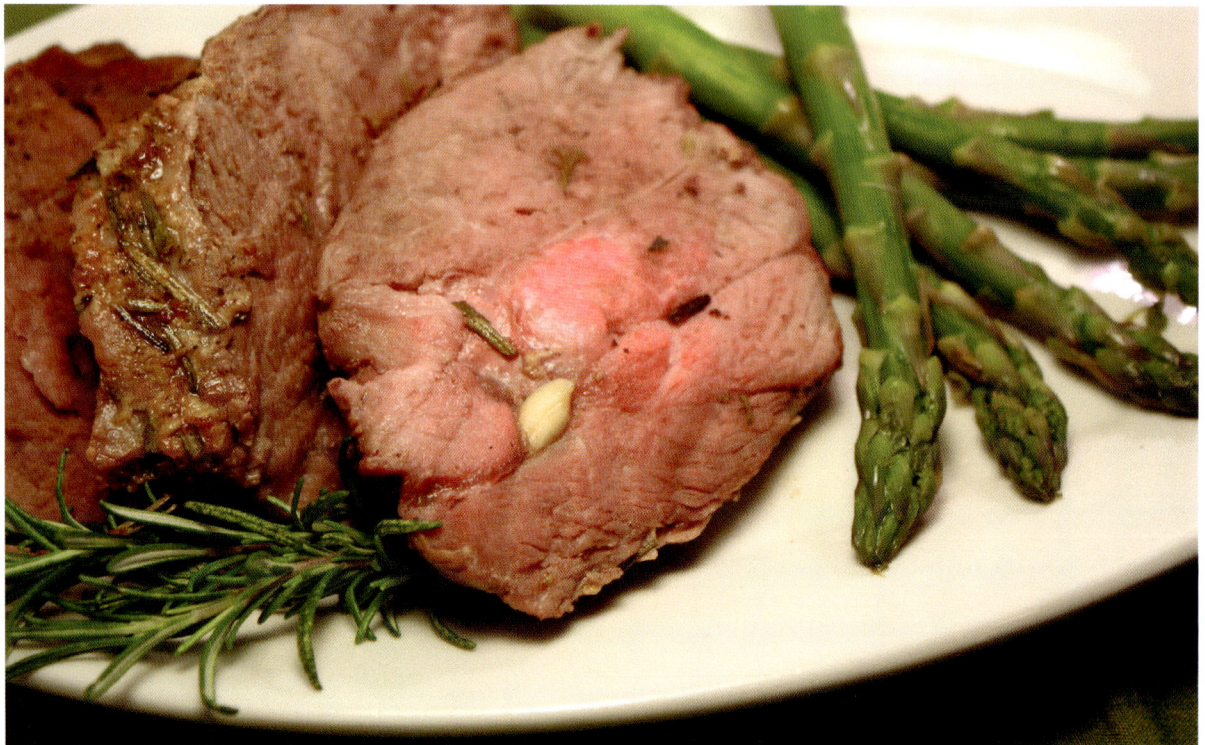

Fennel Pork Loin with Pears

Carnivores will appreciate this dish's amazingly rich and savory flavor, and the cook will certainly appreciate how easy it is to prep and clean up...long live the one-pot dish!

Inspired by *www.realsimple.com*

Serves 4

3 to 4 Tablespoons fennel seeds
4 to 5 cloves garlic, minced
6 Tablespoons olive oil, divided
Salt and pepper to taste
2 pounds boneless pork loin or roast
3 red onions, quartered
3 to 4 firm pears (such as Bartlett), cored and quartered

1. Heat oven to 400 degrees. Mix the fennel, the garlic, 2 tablespoons of oil, salt, and pepper. Rub the mixture over the pork then place the pork in a large roasting pan.
2. In another bowl, mix the onions, pears, salt, pepper, and the remaining oil. Scatter around the pork and roast until cooked through, about 70 minutes. Transfer the pork to a cutting board and let rest 5 minutes before slicing. Serve with the roasted pears and onions.

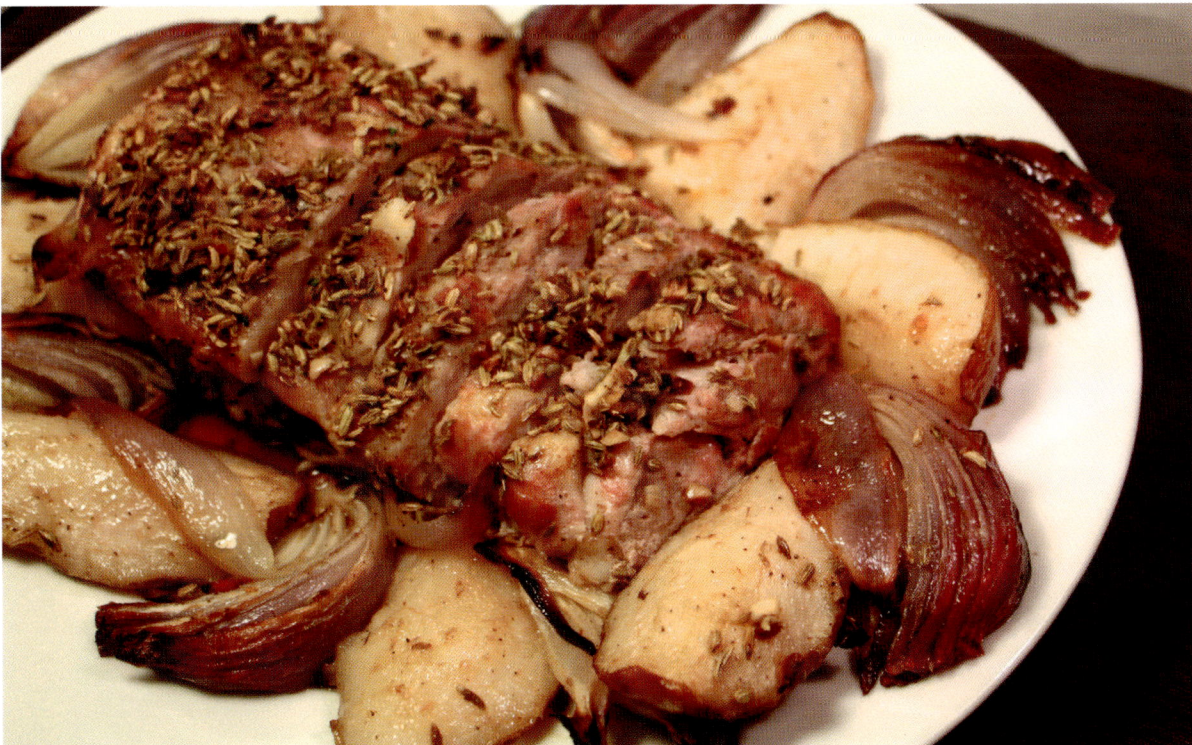

Pistachio Pesto

This unusual pesto makes an excellent accompaniment to basic grilled chicken, steak, lamb, or shrimp. My family's personal favorite is to smother it over pan-grilled steak served alongside broccoli that has been sautéed in the steak juices. Delicious!

Serves 4

> 1/2 cup fresh flat leaf parsley
> 1/4 cup roasted shelled pistachios
> 1 small clove garlic
> 1/4 teaspoon salt
> 1/4 teaspoon pepper
> 1/4 cup plus 2 Tablespoons olive oil

1. In a food processor, finely chop the first five ingredients with 1/4 cup of oil.
2. Drizzle in the remaining olive oil if necessary and serve.

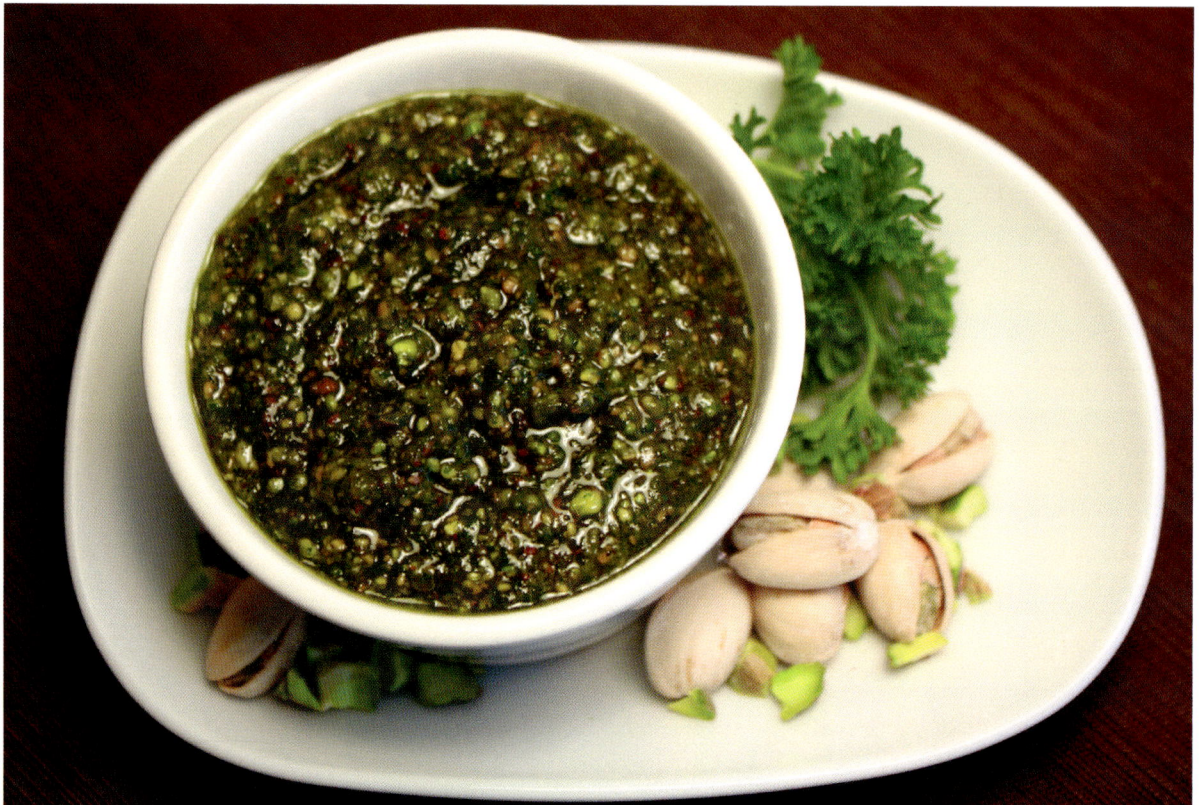

Tropical Burger

I've had a few brief flirtations with vegetarianism, but in the end I just can't give up burgers that taste this yummy. I think you'll enjoy the tropical influences in this dish, but if not, then top it with just the mustard!

Serves 4

> 1-1/2 pounds ground beef or buffalo (at least 80% lean and grass-fed)
> Salt and pepper (optional)
> 1/4 cup mustard
> 1 firm avocado, sliced
> 1/2 small red onion, sliced
> 4 canned pineapple slices
> Chopped cilantro (optional)

1. Divide meat into four equal portions. Form each portion loosely into a 3/4-inch thick patty. Season with salt and pepper, if desired.
2. Grill patties about 5-6 minutes per side.
3. Spread mustard on each patty and top with the avocado, red onions, pineapple, and cilantro.

Tip: Before cooking, make a slight depression with your thumb on each patty. This will help prevent the burger from swelling as it cooks.

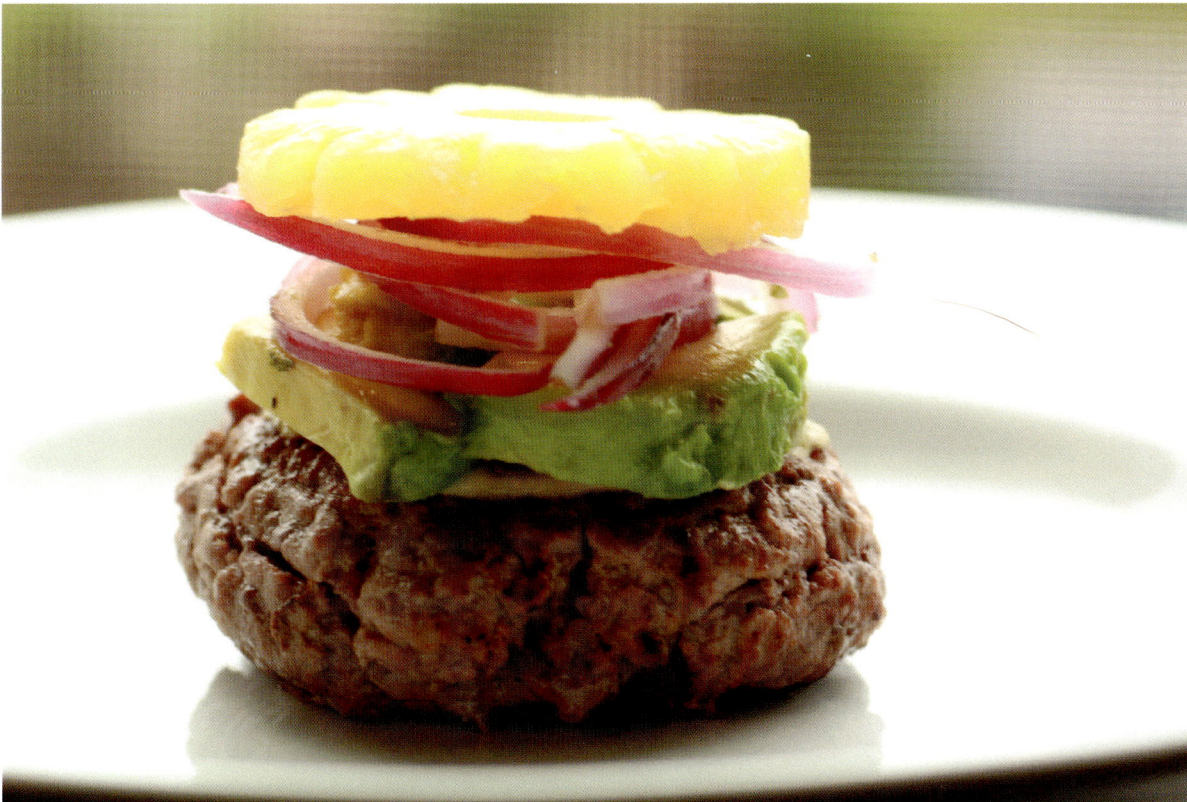

Fish & Seafood

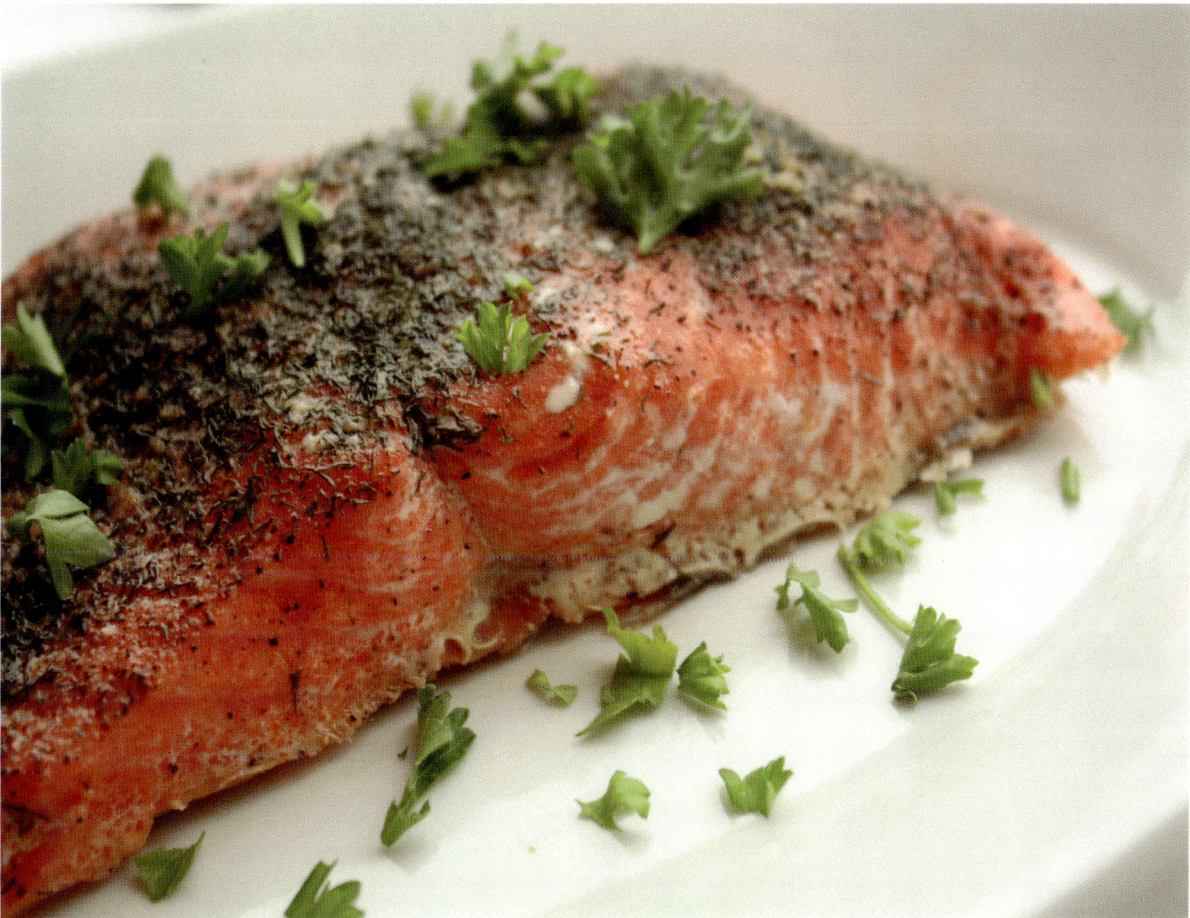

1-2-3 Salmon

Soba Noodle Salmon

Soba noodles are made from buckwheat, which - surprise - contains no wheat! Buckwheat is not a wheat but is a plant in the carrot family, and is low in fat, high in iron, and gluten free. An important note: not all soba noodles are gluten-free! Some are made with a portion of wheat as well as buckwheat, so you have to read the package to ensure that they are 100% buckwheat.

Serves 4

- 1/2 cup carrots, diagonally sliced
- 1/2 cup snow peas
- 3 Tablespoons coconut or olive oil, divided
- Four 6-ounce skinless salmon fillets
- Salt and pepper
- 8 ounces 100% buckwheat soba noodles
- 4 scallions, sliced
- Ginger vinaigrette (see below)
- 2 Tablespoons toasted sesame seeds

1. Sauté carrots and snow peas in 1 tablespoon oil until crisp-tender.
2. Season salmon fillet with salt and pepper. Cook in remaining 2 tablespoons oil in a skillet over medium heat until opaque, 5-6 minutes per side; then flake.
3. Cook 8 ounces soba noodles; rinse.
4. Toss with snow peas, carrots, scallions, and ginger vinaigrette. Top with salmon and sprinkle with sesame seeds.

Ginger Vinaigrette:

- 1/4 cup rice vinegar
- 2 Tablespoons honey or brown rice syrup
- 1 Tablespoon finely grated ginger, or 1 teaspoon dried ginger powder
- 1/4 cup olive oil
- Salt and pepper

1. Whisk all ingredients in a small bowl.
2. Keep covered in the refrigerator if prepared ahead.

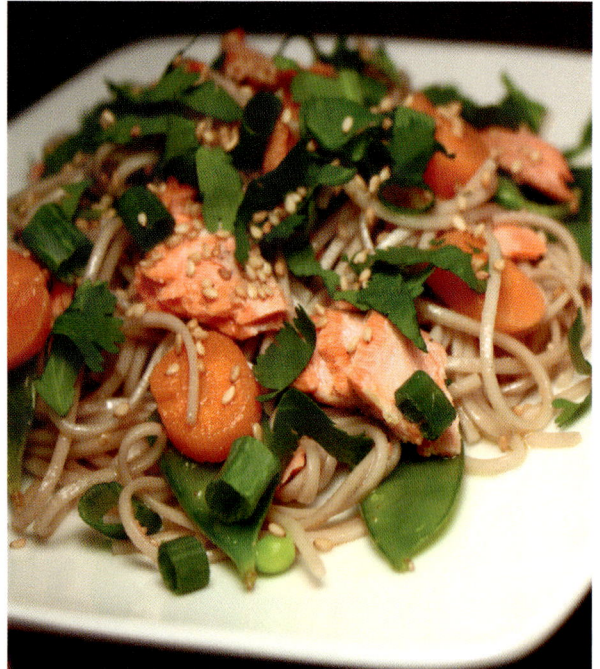

Curried Shrimp with Rice

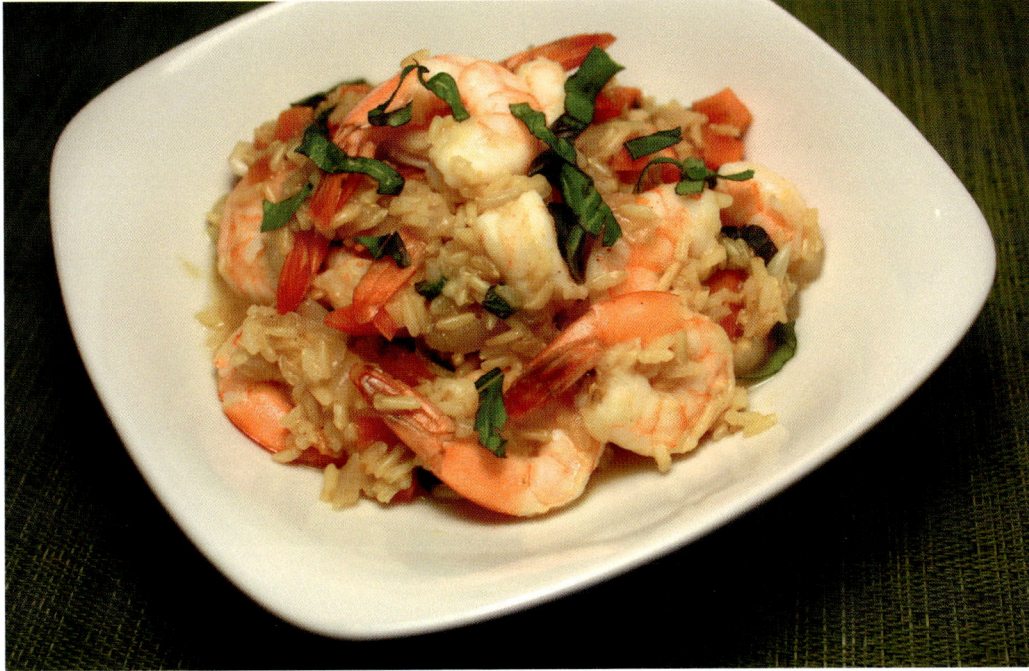

This is one of my many "kitchen staples" recipes - I'm likely to have all of the ingredients on hand in my pantry or freezer without having to make a special trip to the store, so it's a great last minute go-to for lunch or a quick dinner. Simple, quick, and tasty!

Serves 4

- 1 Tablespoon coconut oil
- 1 large onion, chopped
- 3 carrots, chopped
- 3 cloves garlic, chopped
- 3 teaspoons curry powder
- 1 cup long-grain brown rice
- 2-1/2 cups water
- 1/2 teaspoon salt
- 1/2 teaspoon pepper
- 1 to 1-1/2 cup frozen peas, defrosted
- 2 pounds large shrimp, peeled and deveined
- 2/3 cup fresh basil

1. Heat the oil in a large skillet over medium heat. Add the onion and carrots and cook, stirring occasionally, until soft, 6 to 8 minutes.
2. Add the garlic and curry and cook, stirring, until fragrant, 2 minutes.
3. Add the rice, water, salt, and pepper and bring to a boil. Reduce heat to medium low, cover, and simmer for 15 minutes.
4. Stir in peas and nestle shrimp in the partially cooked rice. Cover and cook until the shrimp are opaque throughout, 4 to 5 minutes. Stir in the basil and serve.

Pasta & Shrimp Packets

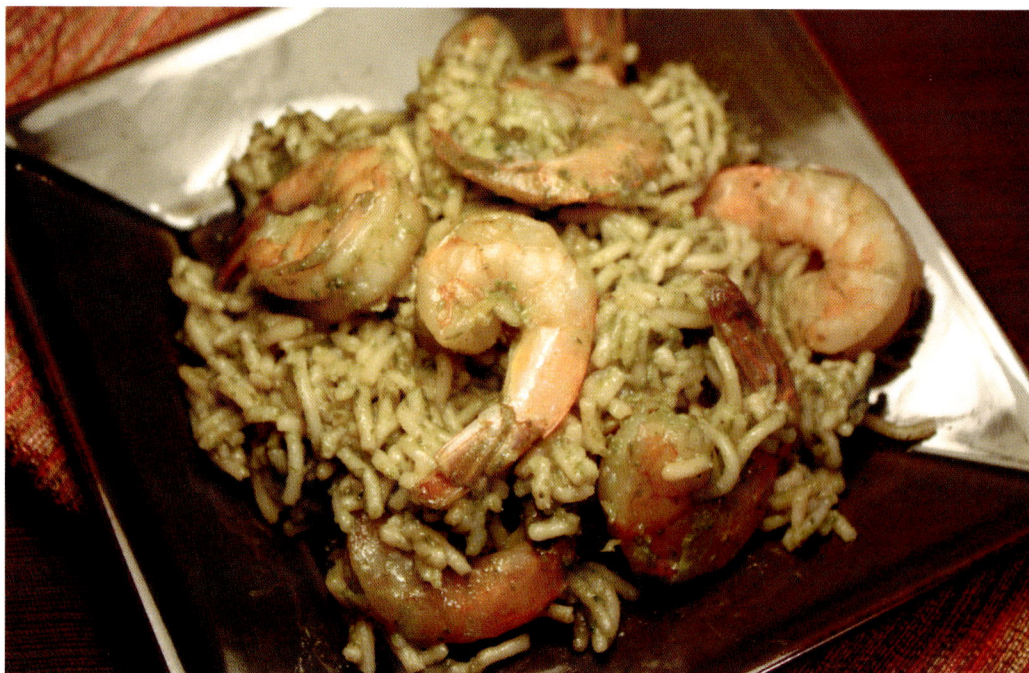

I like to serve this dish for dinner guests when I'd rather spend more time socializing than cooking before the meal. This dish is the ideal solution since the packets can be prepared in advanced and put in the oven when your guests arrive.

Serves 4

4 teaspoons olive oil
1 pound uncooked rice pasta fettuccine or spaghetti
2/3 cup spinach pesto sauce, divided (see Poor Man's Pesto in the Pasta section)
1 pound 10 ounces large raw shrimp, peeled
2 cloves garlic, crushed
Salt and pepper
1/2 cup chicken broth

1. Preheat oven to 425 degrees.
2. Cut out four 12-inch squares of aluminum foil paper. Drizzle 1 teaspoon of olive oil in the center of each square.
3. Cook pasta in lightly salted boiling water for 6 minutes, until just softened. Drain and set aside.
4. Mix together the pasta and half of the pesto sauce. Divide the pasta among the squares. Divide the shrimp and place on top of the pasta.
5. Mix together the remaining pesto sauce and the garlic; spoon over the shrimp. Season each parcel with salt and pepper and sprinkle with the chicken broth (2 tablespoons broth per packet).
6. Fold the foil edges in to wrap as a loose packet. Place the packets on a cookie sheet and bake for 20 minutes. Transfer the packets to individual serving plates and serve.

1-2-3 Salmon

Basic salmon works with a wide variety of flavors. Though dill is probably the herb most commonly associated with salmon, almost any seasoning will do. I'll often substitute thyme or basil for the dill depending on the season, and I'm sure you'll have your own favorite herb that will taste delicious with this very easy, basic recipe! The important thing is not to let salmon dry out, so bake just until it flakes (about 10 minutes for each inch of thickness).

Serves 4

> Four 6-ounce salmon fillets
> 1/4 teaspoon salt
> 1/2 teaspoon pepper
> 1 teaspoon garlic or onion powder
> 2 teaspoon dried dill
> 2 Tablespoon olive oil

1. Preheat oven to 400 degrees.
2. Arrange salmon fillets, skin side down, on a large baking dish or foil-lined pan. Sprinkle fillets with the salt, pepper, garlic powder, and dill. Drizzle over with the olive oil.
3. Bake for 15-25 minutes, until the salmon flakes easily with a fork.

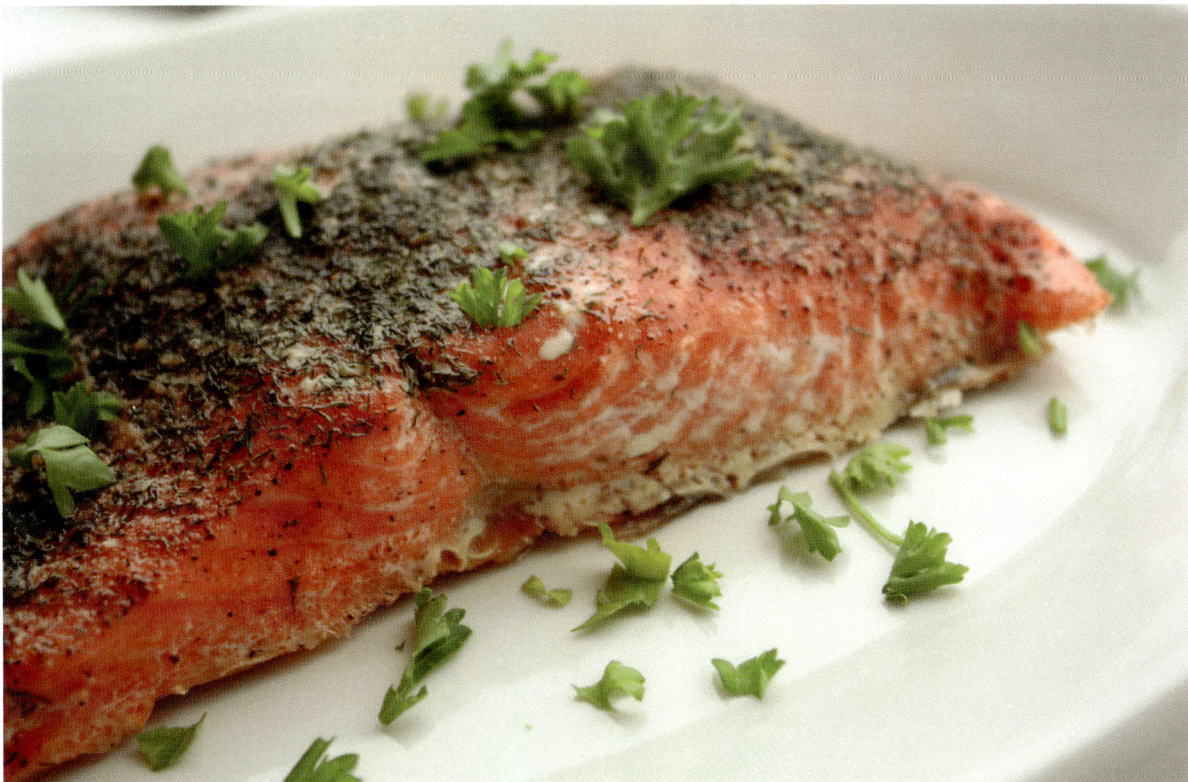

Grilled Mahi-Mahi with Avocado-Melon Salsa

*Jamaican jerk seasoning is a supermarket
staple nowadays, which you'll find easily in the spice aisle. If mahi is unavailable or too pricey at the fish counter, you can readily
substitute thick tilapia fillets (and ditch the grill for a skillet). One final note - I usually double the salsa portion of this recipe so that there are plenty of leftovers for chips and salsa the next day, though this mix is so tasty that often there isn't much left to save!*

Serves 4

> 1 small avocado, diced
> 1 cup 1/3-inch cubes cantaloupe
> 1/2 cup diced red onion
> 1/3 cup chopped fresh cilantro
> Salt and pepper
> 2 Tablespoons coconut oil, divided
> Four 6-ounce mahi-mahi fillets (each about 1 inch thick) or thick tilapia fillets
> 3 Tablespoons Jamaican jerk seasoning
> Homemade tortilla chips (optional, see Chips and Guacamole tortilla chip recipe in
>   the "Snacks" section)

1. Prepare salsa by tossing first 5 ingredients and 1 tablespoon coconut oil in medium bowl to blend.
2. Oil grill or skillet with remaining 1 tablespoon coconut oil and heat to medium-high.
3. Sprinkle the jerk seasoning on both sides of the fish.
4. Grill fish until just opaque in center, about 4 minutes per side. Serve with salsa and tortilla chips.

Tip: This salsa is really at its best when flavored with lime. For non-Elimination Dieters, feel free to replace the oil in the salsa with the shredded zest and juice of 1 large lime. An added benefit is that the acidity of the lime juice keeps the avocado from browning, which means prettier leftover salsa!

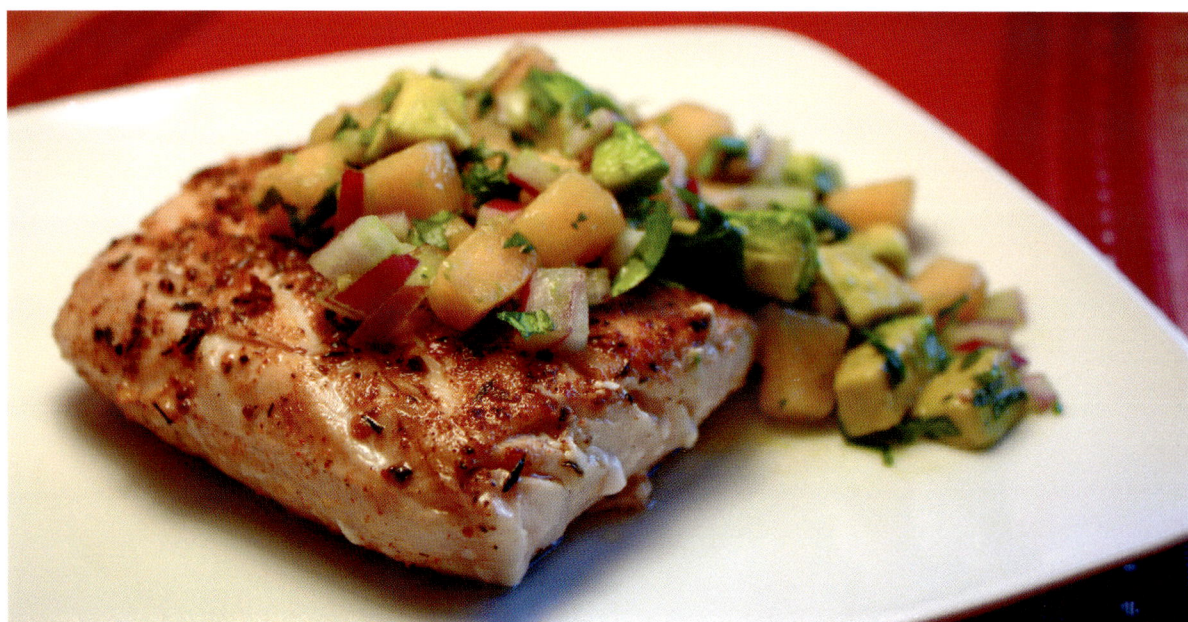

Pasta, Rice & Grains

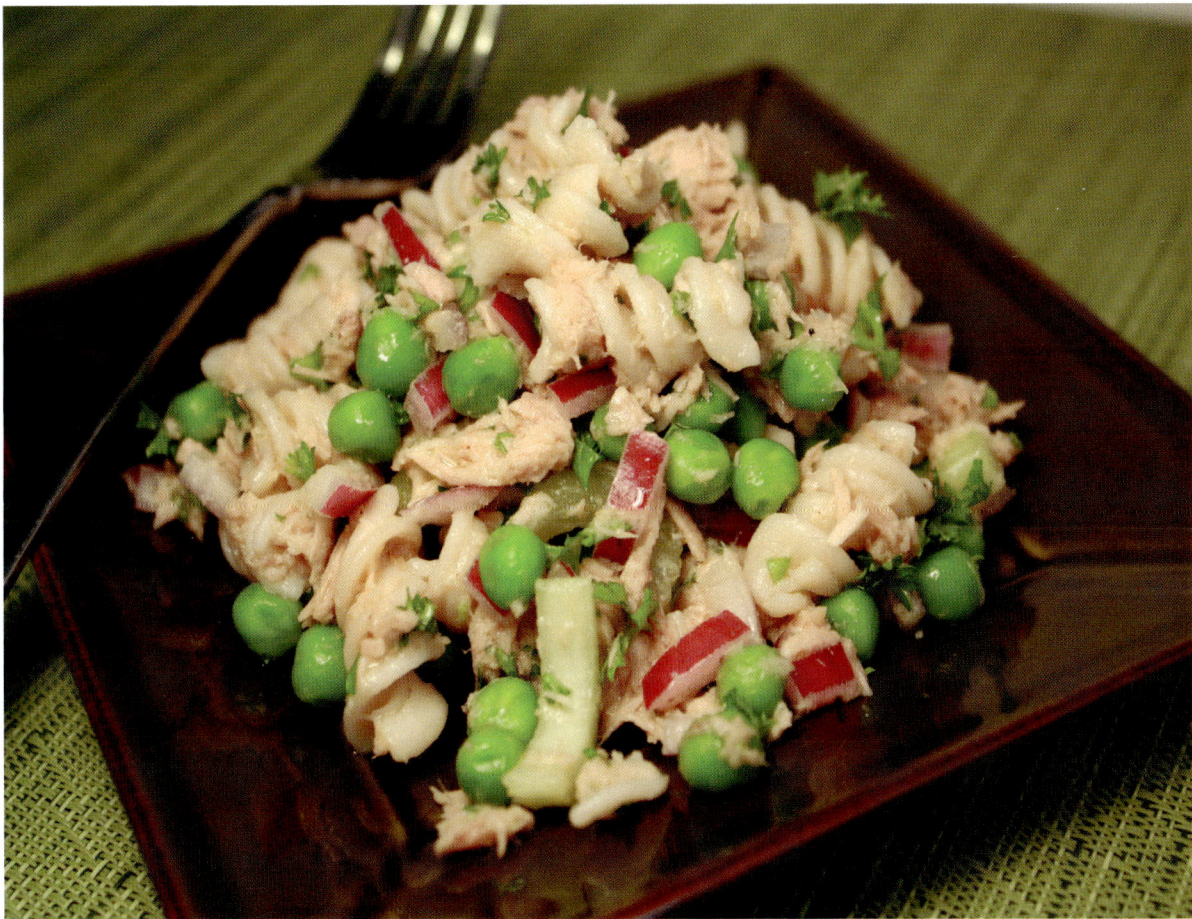

Pea & Tuna Pasta Salad

Creamy Avocado Pasta

Growing up in California, there was never a shortage of avocados on hand to be crafted into creative dishes. This speedy and unique sauce is so creamy, thick, and rich that you'll think there's actual cream hiding somewhere in there!

Serves 2

6-8 ounces rice pasta
8 ounces asparagus, cut into 1-inch pieces
2-3 cloves garlic
2/3 cups olive oil
1 large ripe avocado, pitted and peeled
3/4 to 1 cup basil leaves, densely packed
1/2 teaspoon salt
Pepper

1. Cook pasta according to directions on package.
2. Meanwhile, steam the asparagus until crisp-tender.
3. Make the sauce by blending garlic and olive oil in a blender or food processor. Process until smooth. Add the avocado, basil, and salt. Process until smooth.
4. Add asparagus to the pasta. Pour sauce over the pasta mix and toss until fully coated. Garnish with black pepper.

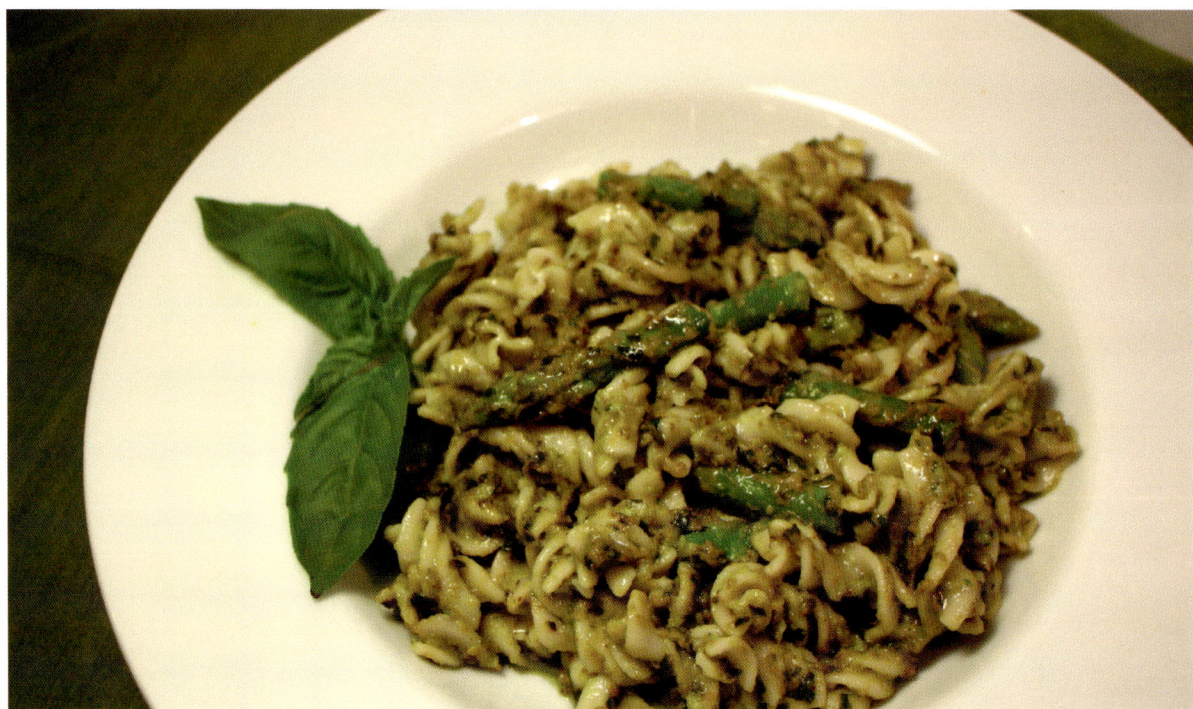

Turkey Bolognese

Think you can't enjoy spaghetti while on the Elimination Diet? Wrong! Beets execute a convincing performance in this mock tomato sauce - so much so that you won't be able to detect any trace of them. Try not to overcook the sauce once the beets are added, as they discolor with excessive cooking. For a vegetarian sauce, simply omit the turkey.

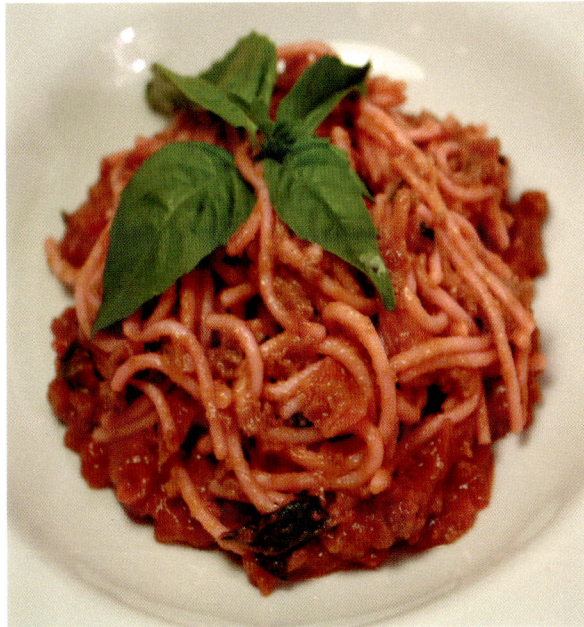

Serves 4 (makes 3 cups)

> 1/2 to 2/3 pounds ground turkey
> 1 large onion, finely chopped
> 3 cloves garlic, finely chopped
> 1/3 cup olive oil
> 1 Tablespoon white or red wine vinegar
> One 8-ounce can beets, drained and the
>   liquid reserved
> One 14- to 15-ounce can pumpkin puree,
>   or 2 cups mashed sweet potatoes
> 1 teaspoon coarse salt
> 1 teaspoon black pepper
> 1/2 cup chopped fresh basil
> 1/2 cups chicken or vegetable broth
> 1 Tablespoon honey
> 1 Tablespoon almond or quinoa flour
> Cooked rice pasta

1. In a large stock pot, sauté the turkey, onion, and garlic in olive oil, breaking the turkey up into small chunks.
2. Add vinegar. Simmer for 5 minutes.
3. Meanwhile, puree beets in blender or food processor until smooth.
4. Add beets, pumpkin puree or sweet potato, salt, pepper, and basil to pan. Stir until combined.
5. Stir in the broth and honey. Simmer over low heat for 5 minutes.
6. Add the flour a bit at a time and stir to combine. Taste and adjust seasoning. If sauce is too thick, add a little more broth to thin.
7. Serve with rice pasta.

Poor Man's Pesto

Pesto is traditionally prepared with basil and pine nuts, but spinach and walnuts taste similar and are both cheaper and easier to find year-round. Pesto is quick, versatile, and adds a great pop of color to bland dishes. Try it drizzled over broiled chicken, fish, or steak for a sophisticated variation on traditional fare.

Serves 4

> 1 pound uncooked rice pasta (fettuccine or spaghetti)
> 1/4 cup walnuts or pine nuts
> 2 cloves garlic
> 1/2 pound baby spinach (about 10 cups)
> 1/3 cup olive oil
> 1/4 teaspoon salt
> 1/4 teaspoon black pepper

1. Cook the pasta according to the package directions. Drain and return it to the pot.
2. Meanwhile, pulse the walnuts and garlic and a food processor or blender until chopped. Add the spinach, oil, salt, and pepper. Puree until smooth, scraping down the sides of the processor bowl as necessary.
3. Add the pesto to the pasta and toss to combine.

Tip: Traditional pesto usually includes parmesan cheese. For non-Elimination Dieters, feel free to add 1/2 cup grated parmesan cheese to this recipe for an extra rich finish.

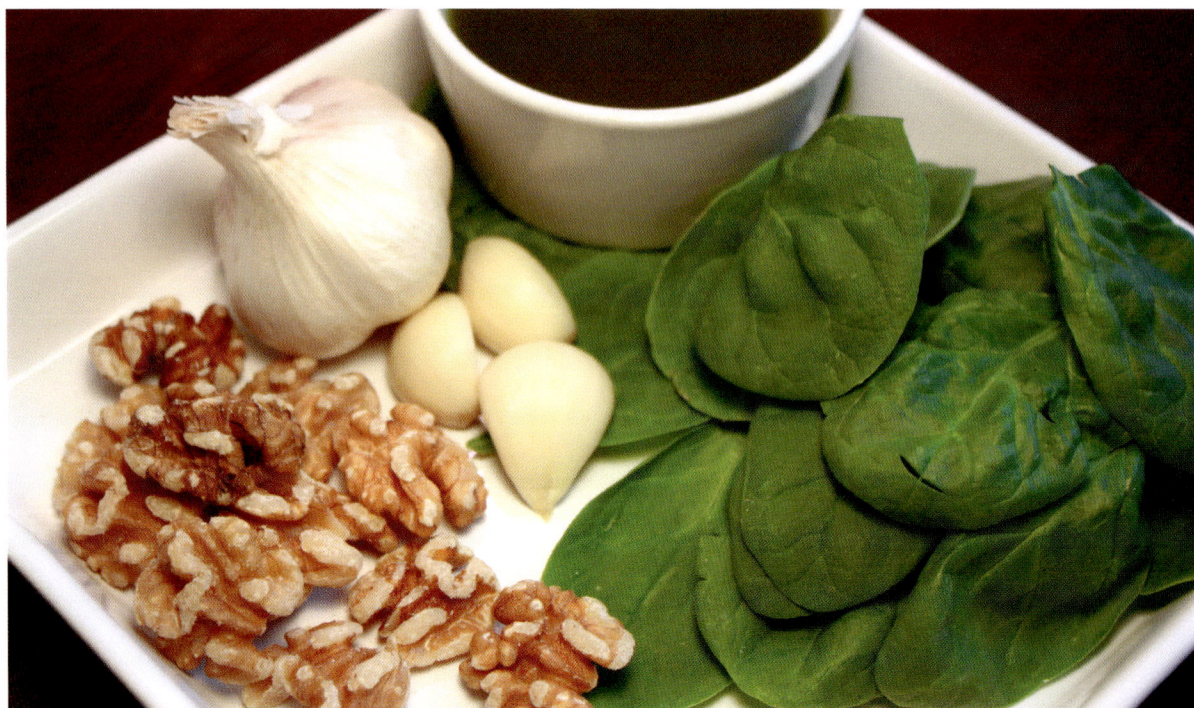

Roasted Butternut Squash & Shallots Pasta

If you have ever considered investing in a quality vegetable peeler, do it! A well-designed peeler makes easy work of stripping difficult skins and saves tons of wrist power - not to mention that it's safer and less time-consuming than using a knife or dull peeler. Try this great pasta dish as a side to chicken or pork, and don't be surprised if it outshines or becomes the main course!

Serves 2

- 3 cups peeled, cubed (about 1 inch) butternut squash
- 1 Tablespoon maple syrup
- 2 Tablespoons olive oil, divided
- 1 teaspoon salt
- 1/2 teaspoon pepper
- 8 shallots, peeled and halved lengthwise (about 1/2 pound)
- 2 Tablespoons chopped fresh or 2 teaspoon dried rubbed sage
- 4 ounces uncooked rice pasta

1. Preheat oven to 475 degrees.
2. Combine squash, maple syrup, 1 tablespoon oil, salt, pepper, and shallots in a large pan and toss well.
3. Bake for 20 minutes or until squash and shallots are tender, stirring occasionally. Stir in sage.
4. While squash mixture bakes, cook pasta according to package directions. Drain. Place cooked pasta in a bowl. Add remaining 1 tablespoon olive oil, toss well.
5. Serve squash mixture over pasta.

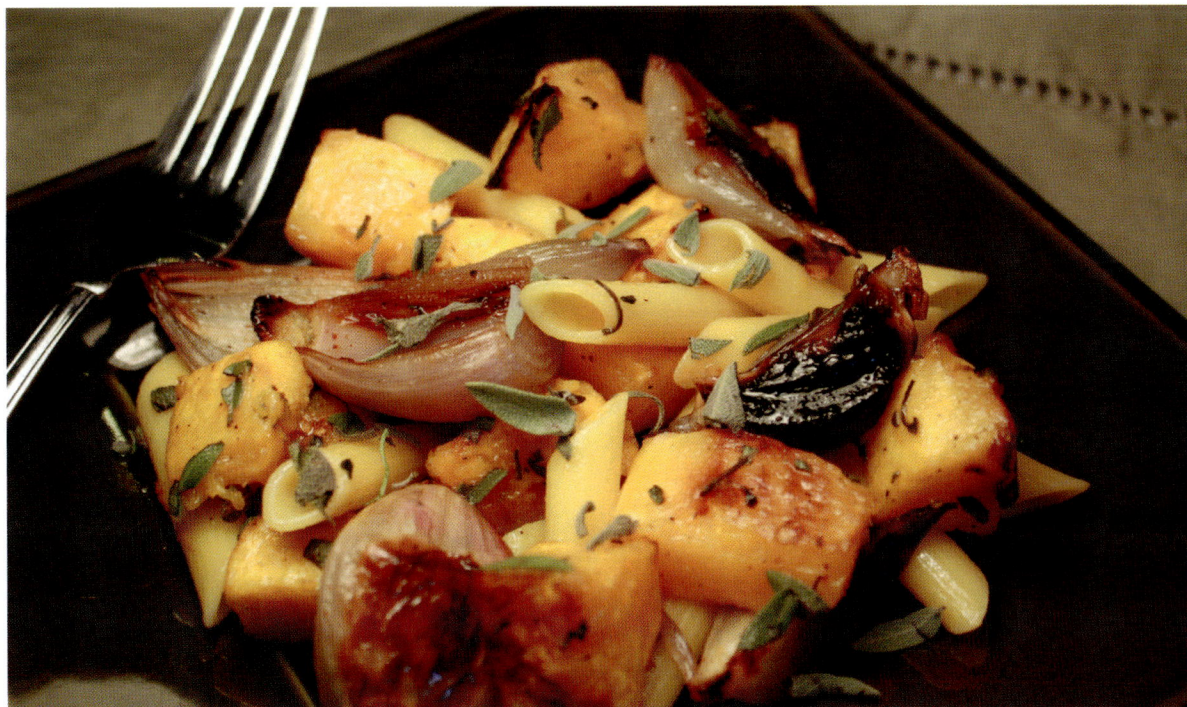

Pea & Tuna Pasta Salad

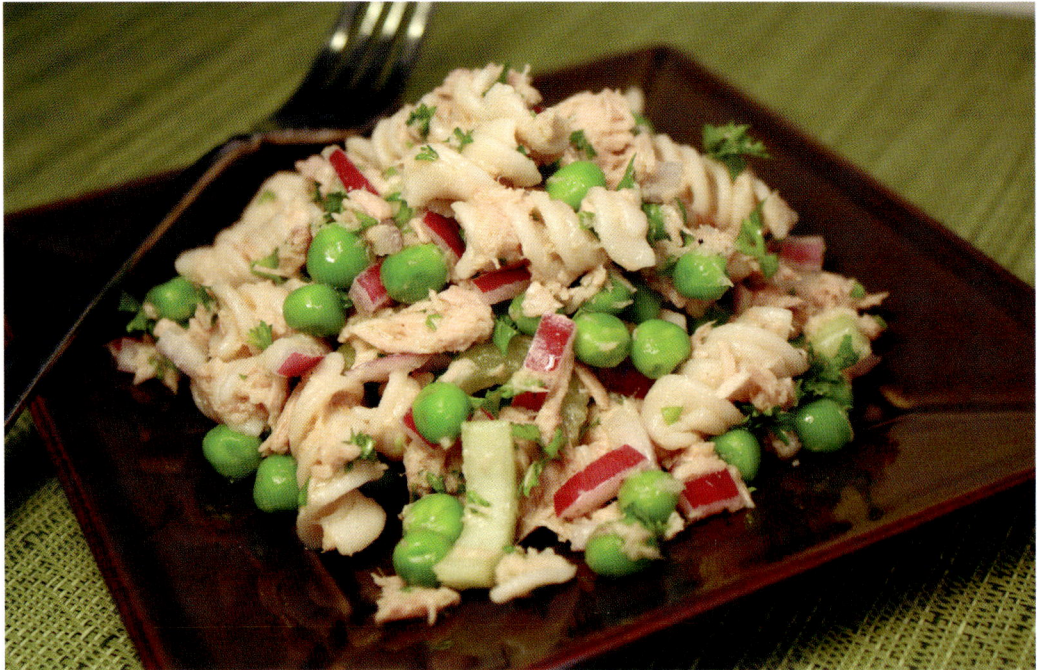

This is your classic "pantry staples" meal, composed of ingredients that you likely already have stocked in your pantry and fridge. It really hits the spot for a light dinner on a warm summer evening, and makes great leftovers for lunch the next day.

Adapted from *www.realsimple.com*

Serves 4

4 cups uncooked spiral rice pasta
2 stalks celery, chopped
2 cups frozen peas, thawed
1/2 red onion, chopped
1/2 cup parsley, chopped
Three 6-ounce cans tuna, drained

Dressing:

1/2 cup olive oil
1/3 cup red wine vinegar
1 teaspoon spicy mustard
2 teaspoon salt
1/2 teaspoon pepper

1. Cook the pasta according to package directions. Drain and rinse under cold running water.
2. In a large bowl, combine the pasta, celery, peas, onion, parsley, and tuna.
3. Prepare dressing a small bowl by whisking together the five ingredients.
4. Dress salad with dressing and gently toss. Serve at room temperature.

Wild Rice a lá California

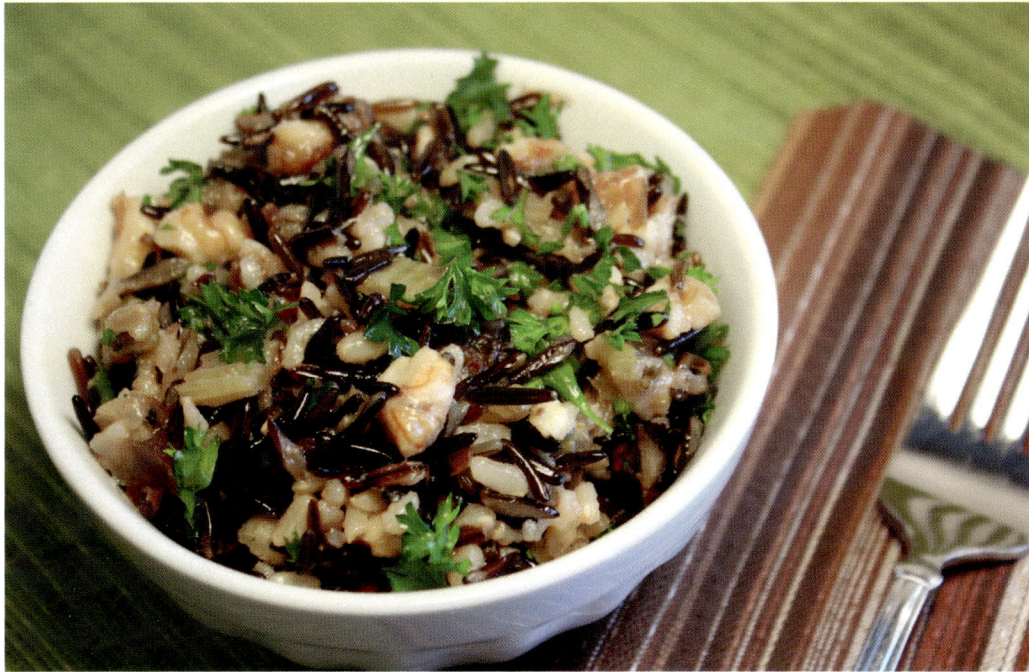

This savory dish reminds me of my childhood growing up in California, which is one of the world's largest producers of dates and nuts. This excellent pilaf-style side dish can be served alongside just about any main meat dish and vegetable, but I tend to favor roasted chicken or lightly seasoned grilled fish with asparagus (another California bounty).

Inspired by *www.bettycrocker.com*

Serves 6

> 2 cups chopped celery (4 stalks)
> 1/2 cup chopped onion
> 1 teaspoon dried thyme (optional)
> 1 Tablespoon olive oil
> 1 cup wild rice, rinsed and drained
> 2 cups chicken or vegetable broth
> 1 cup water
> 1/2 cup parsley, chopped
> 1/2 cup pitted whole dates, chopped
> 1/2 cup chopped walnuts or almonds, toasted

1. In a large skillet cook the celery, onion, and thyme (if used) in hot olive oil for about 10 minutes or until tender but not brown.
2. Add the uncooked wild rice. Cook and stir for 3 minutes more.
3. Slowly add chicken broth and water. Bring to a boil; reduce heat. Cover and simmer for 50-60 minutes or till rice is tender and most of the liquid is absorbed.
4. Stir in the parsley, dates, and walnuts. Cook, uncovered, for 3-4 minutes more or untill heated through and remaining liquid is absorbed.

Asparagus Risotto

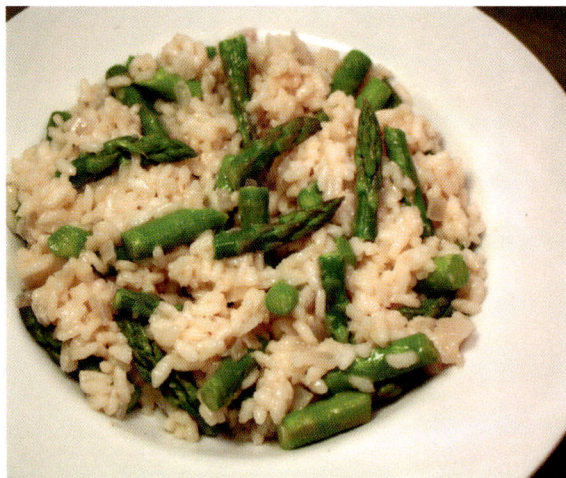

Making risotto at home is easy and healthy! Risotto needs to be stirred frequently, so take the opportunity to multi-task and work on another meal alongside the stove - I like to prep my family's bag lunches for the next day or wash dishes in-between stirring.

Serves 4

3 Tablespoons olive oil, divided
4 scallions or 1/2 red onion, chopped
3/4 cup Arborio rice
3 cups vegetable or chicken broth, hot
1 pound asparagus, cut ends trimmed and cut into 2-inch piece segments

1. In a large pot, heat 2 tablespoons olive oil. Add scallions and Arborio rice. Cook for 3 minutes, stirring, until fragrant.
2. In 3 batches, stir in hot broth 1 cup at a time and cook, stirring frequently, until each is absorbed and rice is "al dente," about 20 minutes. Add hot water if more liquid is needed.
3. Add asparagus and remaining 1 tablespoon olive oil. Cook another 5 minutes until asparagus is tender-crisp.

Tri-Grain Pilaf

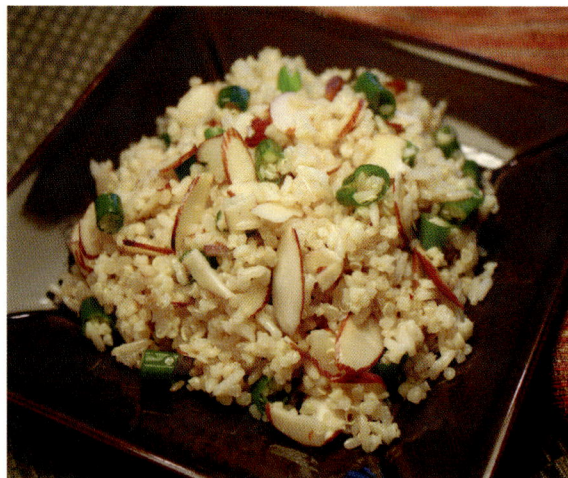

This dish long ago replaced my standard "starch" (as in the protein-vegetable-starch "complete meal" dogma). It's easy, inexpensive, and incredibly versatile - I dare you to find a main course that can't be improved or complemented by the addition of this side dish!

Serves 4

2 Tablespoons olive oil
1/2 cup finely chopped green onions
1 cup uncooked brown basmati or jasmine rice
1/2 cup uncooked quinoa
1/2 cup uncooked millet
3 cups chicken or vegetable broth
1/4 teaspoon salt

1. Heat olive oil in a large nonstick skillet over medium heat. Add onions; cook 2 minutes.
2. Add rice, quinoa, and millet; cook 3 minutes, stirring frequently.
3. Stir in broth and salt. Bring to a boil; cover, reduce heat, and simmer 25 minutes.
4. Remove from heat, fluff with a fork, and serve.

Creamy Rice & Spinach Casserole

This excellent casserole is very flexible, so use your imagination - feel free to substitute chard, carrots, or mushrooms for the spinach - anything you have in the fridge will do. It reheats very well, so it makes for great leftover lunches!

Serves 6

- 4 cloves garlic, minced
- 1 medium to large onion, chopped
- 3-4 Tablespoons olive oil
- 3-4 Tablespoons quinoa flour
- 2 cups almond or rice milk (unsweetened)
- 1 cup vegetable or chicken broth
- Salt and pepper
- One 10-ounce package frozen chopped spinach, thawed and drained, or 1-2 bunches fresh spinach (about 10 ounces)
- 4 cups cooked brown rice

1. Preheat oven to 350 degrees.
2. In a large pot, sauté garlic and onion in olive oil until softened. Sprinkle with flour and stir until mixture is pasty.
3. Slowly add milk and broth. Cook, stirring, at a low boil until sauce thickens. Season with salt and pepper.
4. Remove from heat and stir in spinach and rice (add just enough rice so that mixture is still creamy but not dry).
5. Bake in a greased 9x13 pan for about 30 minutes, until bubbly.

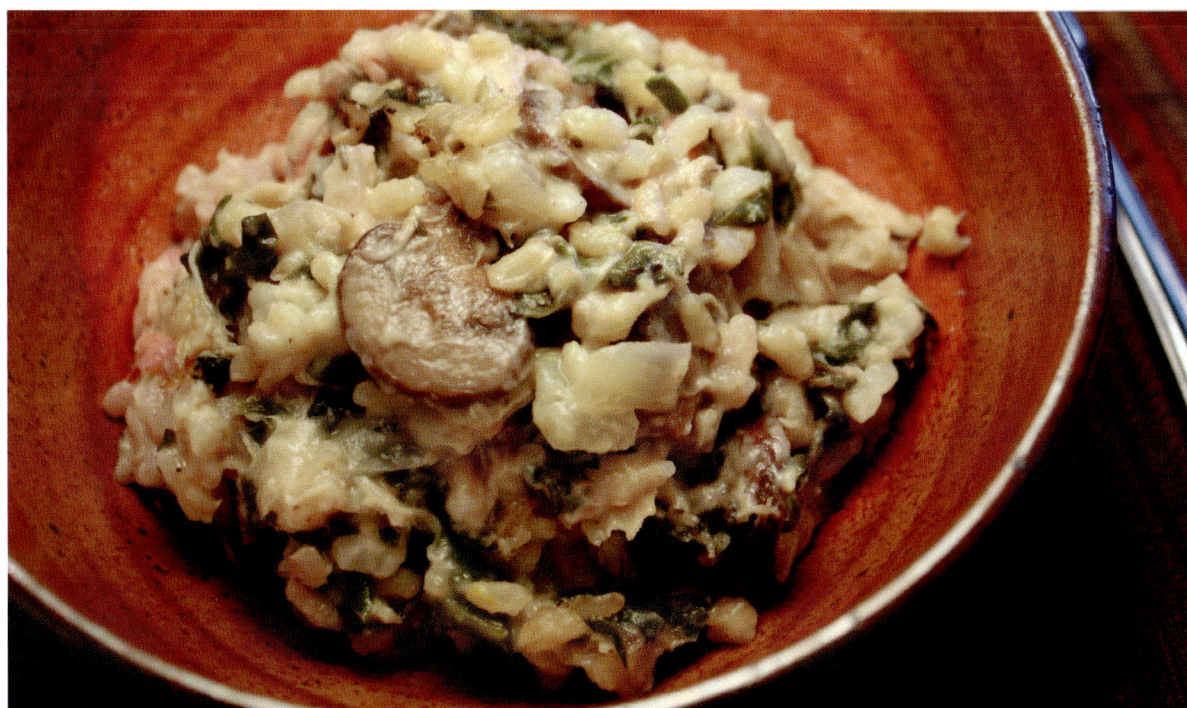

Brown Rice & Bean Salad

The simple Italian dressing in this recipe is quite versatile and can be used throughout the Elimination Diet for all the salads you prepare. Here, it blends with rice and beans to create a lovely summer-appropriate salad for dining al fresco.

Serves 4

2 cups cooked brown rice, cooled
1 can (16 ounces) kidney beans, rinsed and drained
1 medium red onion, chopped
2 large celery stalks, chopped
2 cloves garlic, minced
2 Tablespoons fresh parsley, minced or
2 teaspoons dried parsley flakes
1/4 teaspoon salt
1/4 teaspoon pepper
1/2 cup Italian dressing (see recipe below)

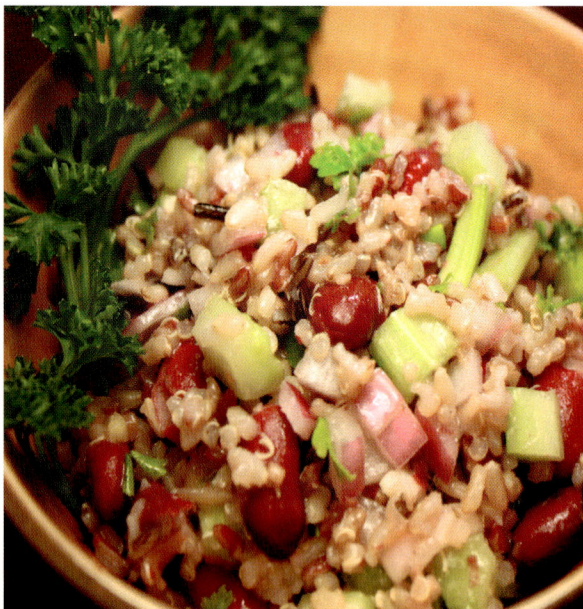

1. In a large bowl, combine the first 8 ingredients. Add enough dressing to lightly coat the mixture, and toss.
2. Cover and refrigerate until cold.

Homemade Italian dressing:
Makes 1 cup

3/4 cups olive oil
1/4 cup white wine vinegar
1 small clove garlic, minced
1/2 teaspoon dried oregano
1/2 teaspoon dried basil
1 teaspoon dried parsley
Salt and pepper to taste

1. Place all the ingredients in a blender and mix for about 10 seconds or until fully combined.
2. Transfer to a glass jar and let stand for 30 minutes to let the flavors meld. Whisk or shake immediately before using.

Vegetables

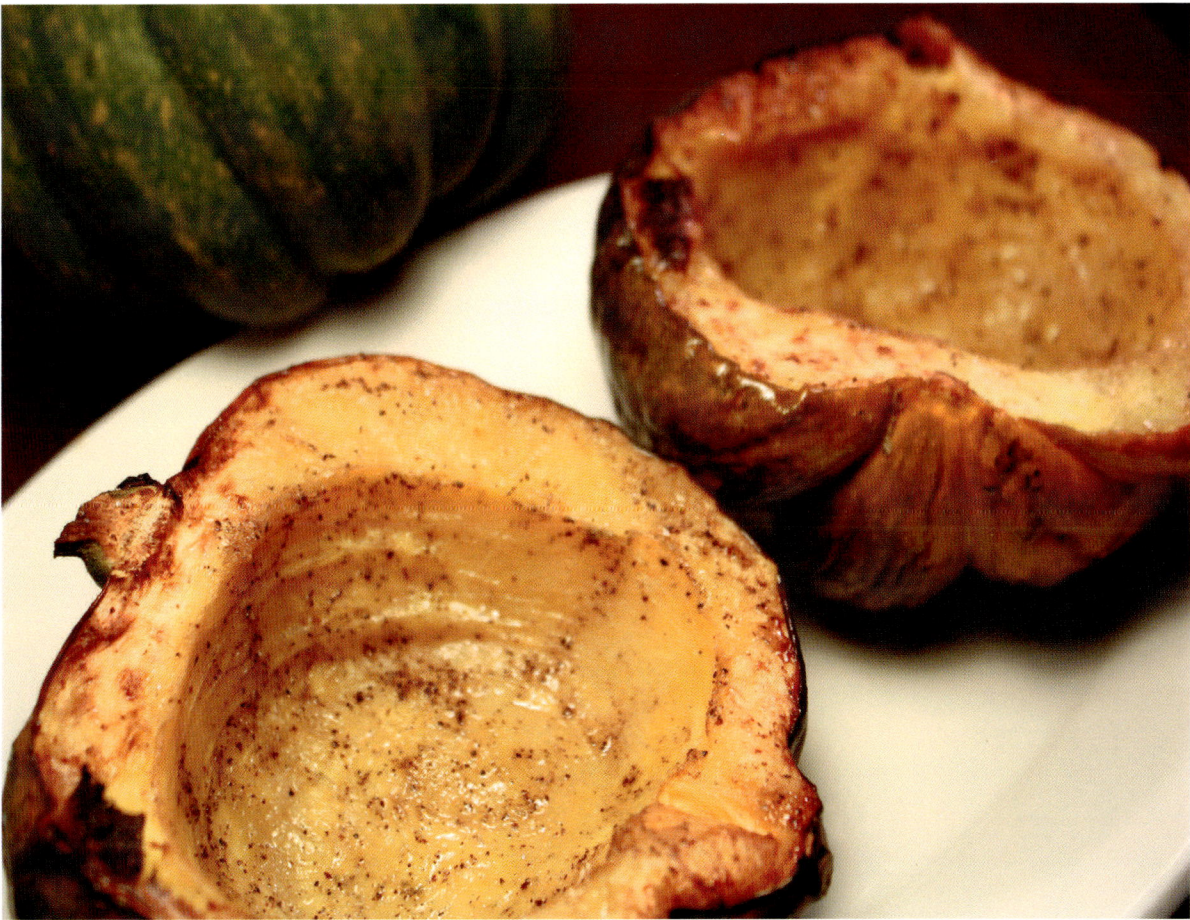

Roasted Acorn Squash

Lentils with Spinach

Lentils are a wonderful dried bean - they're cheap, don't need presoaking, and absorb the flavors of the seasonings they are cooked with. This dish is the perfect embodiment of "the whole is greater than the sum of its parts" concept. Try it and I'm sure you will agree.

Adpated from *www.marthastewart.com*

Serves 4

4 cups water
1/2 cup dried brown lentils
1-1/2 cups carrots, finely chopped
1-1/2 cup onion, finely chopped
2 cloves garlic, minced
1-2 dried bay leaves
Salt and pepper
2 Tablespoons olive oil
8 ounces baby spinach leaves, or whole spinach leaves torn into 1-inch pieces

1. In a large saucepan, combine the water, lentils, carrots, onion, garlic, and bay leaf. Season with salt and pepper. Bring to a boil. Lower the heat and simmer, partially covered, until the lentils are soft, 15-20 minutes. Drain, discarding bay leaf.
2. Add oil, and return pan to medium heat. Stir in the lentils mixture and add spinach. Cook, stirring occasionally, until the spinach is wilted, about 2 minutes. Taste, and adjust for seasoning. Use a slotted spoon to transfer to serving bowls.

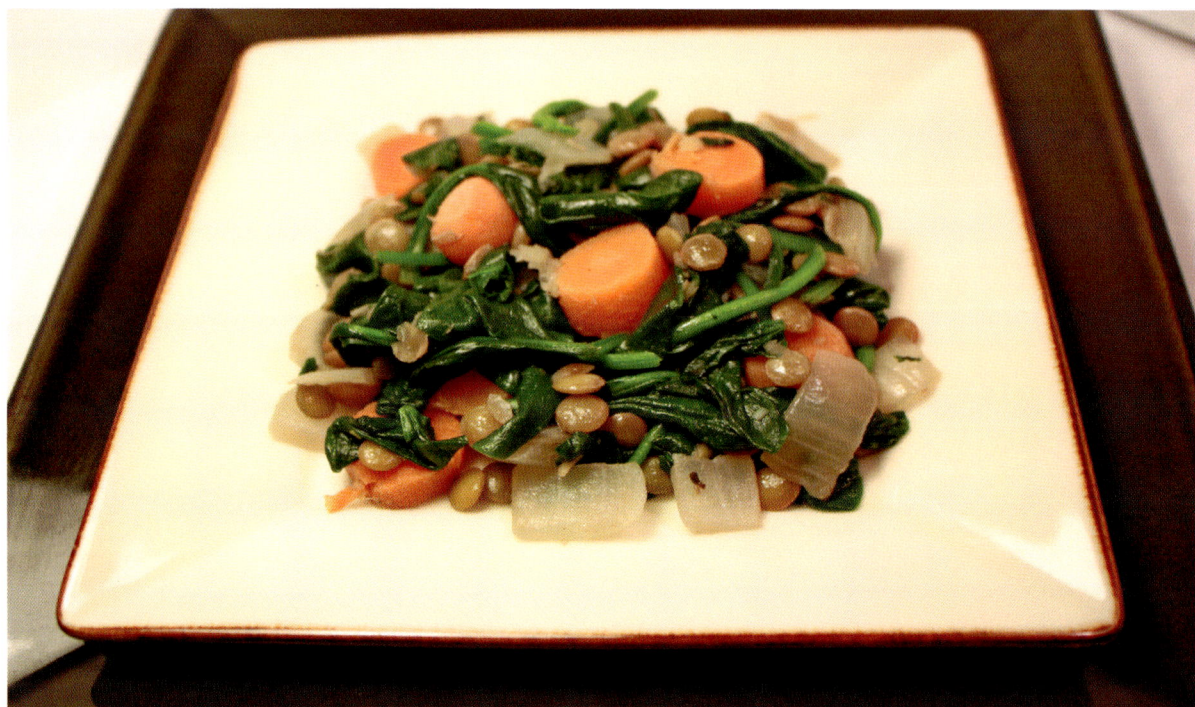

Roasted Brussels Sprouts

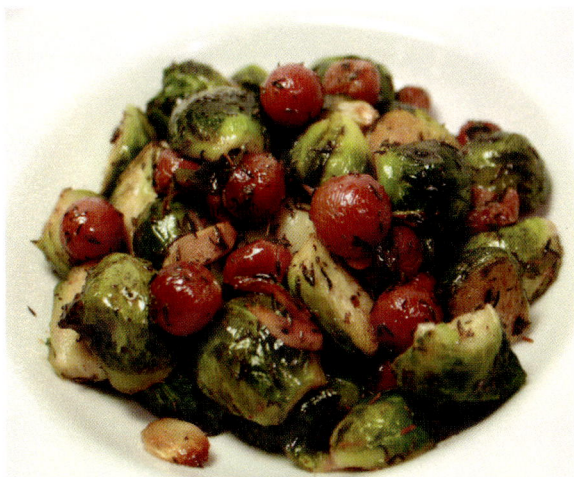

Think you don't like Brussels sprouts? Even naysayers will fall in love with this unexpectedly delicious pairing of grapes and caramelized sprouts! This is a nifty holiday dish, but so delicious that it's sure to make repeat appearances at your dinner table throughout the year.

Serves 6

> 2 pounds Brussels sprouts, trimmed and halved
> 1-1/2 pounds red seedless grapes
> 3 Tablespoons olive oil
> 3 cloves garlic, thinly sliced
> 2 Tablespoons fresh thyme leaves
> Salt and black pepper
> 1 cup pecan halves, toasted (optional)

1. Preheat oven to 375 degrees.
2. In a 9x13 pan, toss the Brussels sprouts and grapes with the oil, garlic, thyme, and salt and pepper to taste.
3. Roast until golden brown and tender, 20 to 25 minutes, shaking the pan after 10 minutes to evenly cook contents.
4. If desired, stir in pecans and serve.

Wilted Lettuce & Peas

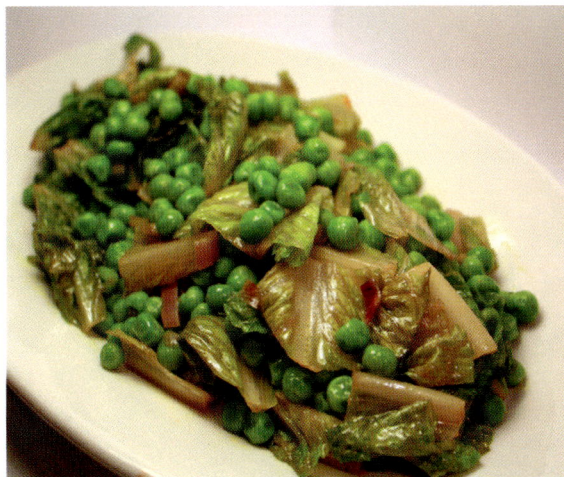

This is such a clever way to utilize lettuce that has seen better days - it becomes sweet and chewy, yet maintains its lovely bright green hue...not to mention the boost of anti-inflammatory and other cancer-fighting properties found in turmeric! Try it alongside simple grilled fish or chicken and congratulate yourself for elevating standard refrigerator staples to a surprisingly novel and healthy side dish!

Serves 3-4

> 1 Tablespoon olive oil
> 2 Tablespoons minced shallots
> 3 cups coarsely chopped romaine lettuce
> 1-1/2 cups frozen peas, thawed
> 1/8 to 1/4 teaspoon turmeric (optional)
> Salt and pepper

1. Heat olive oil in a large skillet over medium heat. Add shallots and cook, stirring frequently, for 4 minutes or until soft.
2. Add lettuce, peas and turmeric; cook for 3 minutes, stirring frequently, or until lettuce is wilted and peas are warm. Season to taste with salt and pepper.

Winter Squash & Black Bean Sauté

Hearty beans, tender squash and caramelized shallots combine to create a simple, comforting dish. Try this with different types of squash as they appear in the market - you'll be pleasantly surprised by how different varieties create totally unique flavors!

Serves 4

> 1 medium-sized winter squash, such as butternut or kabocha
> 2 Tablespoons olive oil
> 3 shallots, halved and sliced
> 1/4 cup chicken stock
> 1-1/2 cups cooked black beans
> Salt and pepper

1. Halve, peel and seed squash. Cut into bite-sized pieces and set aside.
2. Heat olive oil in a large skillet over medium heat. Add shallots and cook, stirring, until slightly softened, about 3 minutes. Add squash, stirring to coat. Add chicken stock, cover, and cook until squash is tender, about 20 minutes.
3. Gently stir in beans and season with salt and pepper to taste. Cook until beans are hot, about 5 minutes. Serve hot or at room temperature.

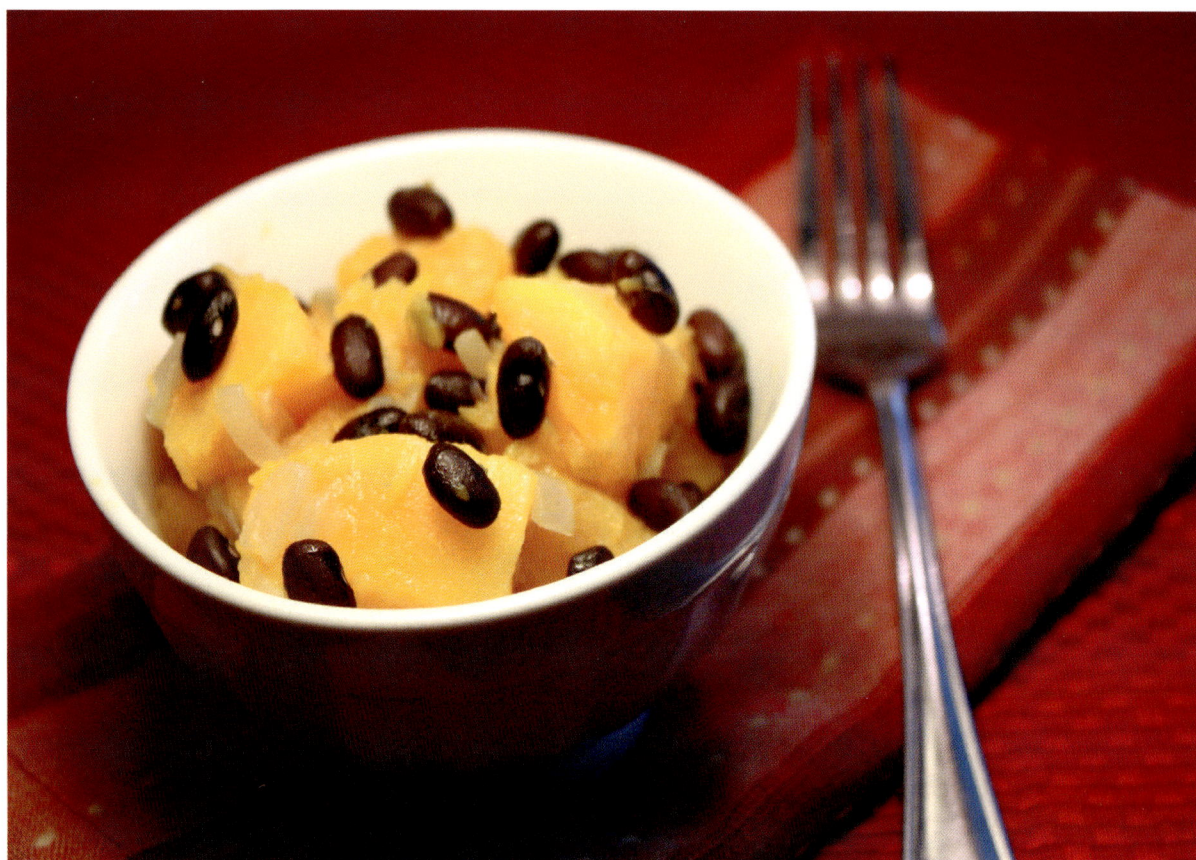

Roasted Beets

Roasting concentrates beets' sweetness and creamy texture. Beets contain abundant nutrients - particularly folate, potassium, and fiber - as do their greens, so don't discard them! Trim greens from the beets after bringing them home (they draw out moisture), leaving an inch or two of stem, then sauté the greens as you would chard or spinach.

Serves 2

2 large beets, each half diced into approximately 8 pieces
2 Tablespoons olive oil, plus extra to garnish
1/2 cup walnuts, toasted
2 Tablespoons parsley, chopped

1. Preheat oven to 400 degrees.
2. Toss beets with olive oil. Place on a baking sheet and bake until tender throughout, 45-60 minutes.
3. Combine the cooked beets with the walnuts and parsley. Serve warm and garnish with olive oil.

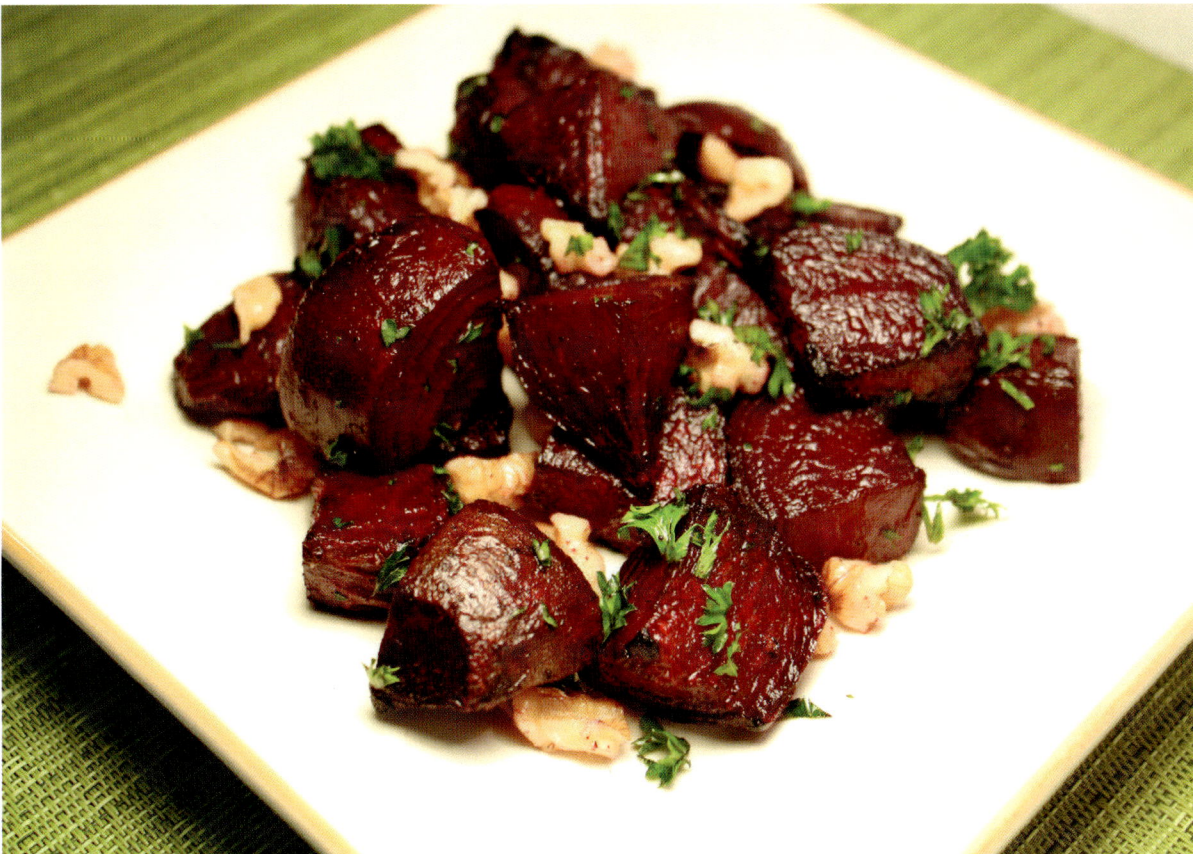

Broccoli Quinoa Pilaf

This tasty side dish easily converts to a main course with the addition of some shredded chicken or turkey. Either way, it's a great option for those who don't love broccoli since the dates and almonds add a sweet and crunchy element that tones down that unique "broccoli flavor."

Inspired by *www.realsimple.com*

Serves 4

3 teaspoons olive oil, divided
1/2 small onion, chopped
3/4 teaspoon salt, plus more to taste
1/4 teaspoon black pepper, plus more
   to taste
1 cup quinoa, rinsed well
1-1/2 cups chicken or vegetable broth
2 cups chopped broccoli
1/4 cup chopped dates
1/2 cup roasted almonds, coarsely
chopped or 1/3 cup slivered almonds,
toasted
2 scallions, sliced

1. Heat 1 teaspoon of the oil in a medium saucepan over medium-high heat. Add the onion, salt, and pepper. Cook, stirring occasionally, until softened and starting to brown, 3-4 minutes.
2. Add the quinoa and broth to the saucepan and bring to a boil; reduce heat to low, cover, and simmer gently until almost all the water has evaporated, 10-12 minutes. Add the broccoli and dates into the quinoa, cover, and cook until the quinoa and broccoli are tender, 8-10 minutes more. Remove from heat and stir in the remaining 2 teaspoons olive oil, almonds, scallions, and season with salt and pepper.

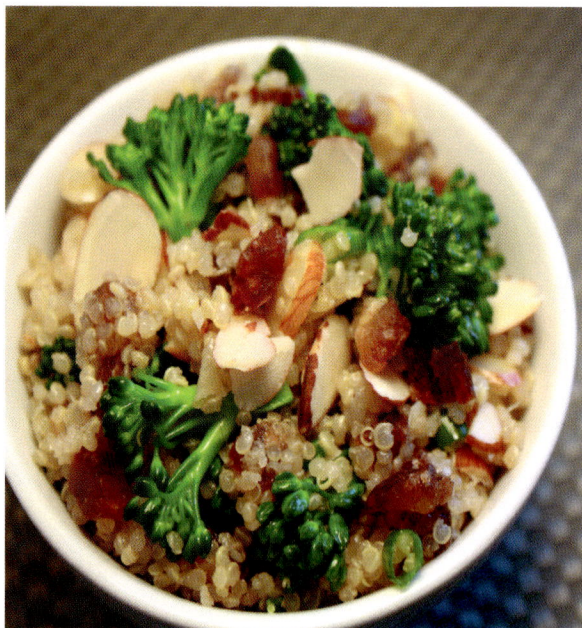

Millet & Cauliflower "Mashed Potatoes"

Craving mashed potatoes? Here's your fix! This awesome faux potato trick was sent to me by my sister-in-law, who is a fantastic cook and has all sort of culinary tricks up her sleeve....

Adapted from *The Self-Healing Cookbook* by Kristina Turner
Courtesy of Christi Lehner-Collins at *www.bostonhealthcoach.com*

Serves 6

3 cups water or vegetable broth
1 cup millet
1 head cauliflower, chopped
Salt and pepper to taste

1. Put the water, millet, and cauliflower in a pot of water on the stove to boil.
2. Once water boils, reduce heat and simmer the mixture until the water is all absorbed (about 20-25 minutes).
3. Once the millet mixture is done, puree in a food processor or with a hand blender until smooth.
4. Add salt and pepper to taste.

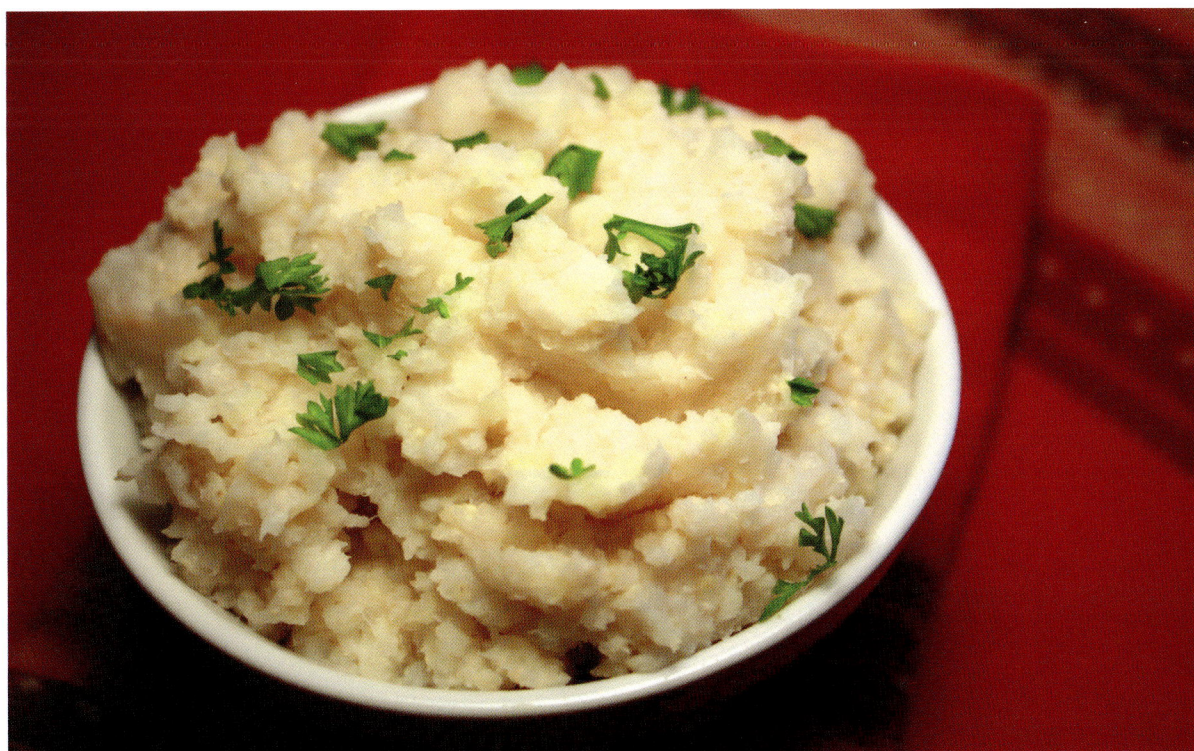

Spaghetti Squash with Mushrooms & Herbs

Tired of pasta? Spaghetti squash is a great and healthy substitute that packs a ton of fiber, vitamins, and texture. Give it a try!

Serves 4

One 2-1/2-pound spaghetti squash, halved lengthwise and seeds discarded
3 Tablespoons olive oil, divided
Salt and pepper
1/2 cup finely chopped onions
2 cups thinly sliced mushrooms
1/4 cup minced fresh parsley leaves
2 Tablespoons minced fresh chives

1. Preheat oven to 350 degrees.
2. In the cavity of each squash, spread 1 tablespoon oil and sprinkle with salt and pepper. Place the squash cut-side down on a greased, foil-lined baking sheet.
3. Bake for 30-45 minutes.
4. Meanwhile, sauté onions and mushrooms in the remaining 1 tablespoon olive oil until brown.
5. Remove squash from the oven and scrape out squash meat with a fork to create shreds.
6. Toss the squash shreds with the mushroom sauté, parsley, chives, and salt and pepper to taste.

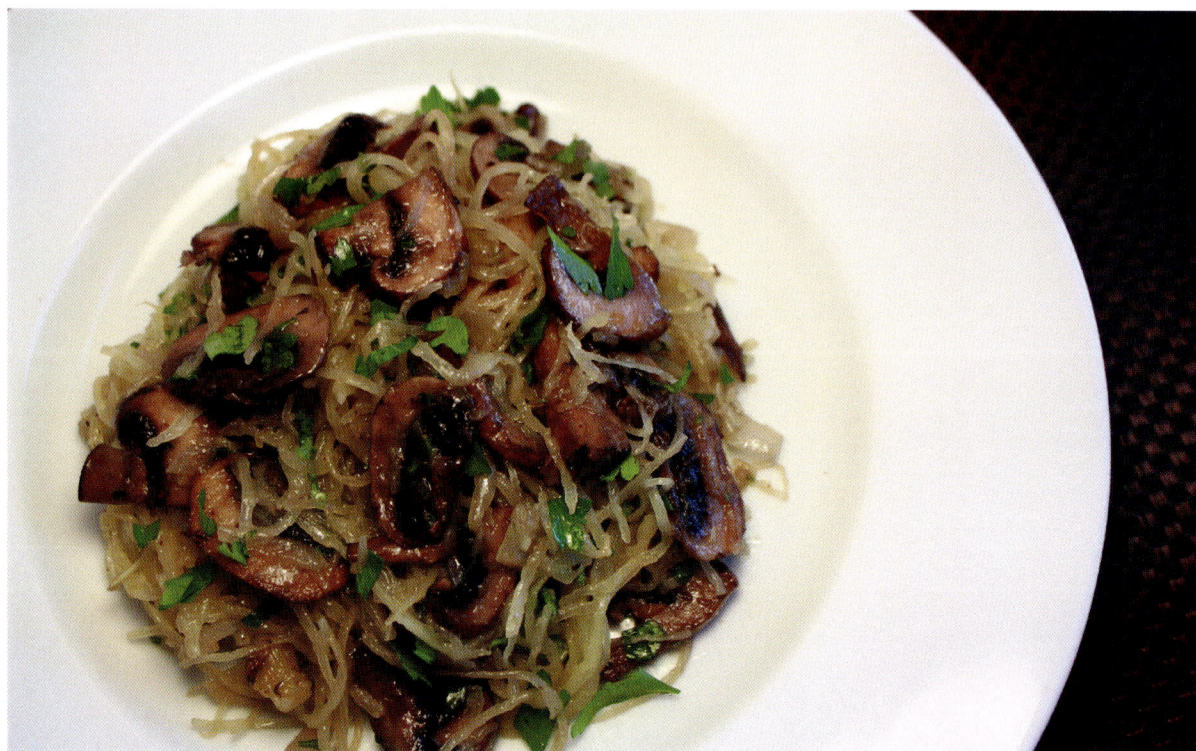

Roasted Acorn Squash

Acorn squash are ridiculously easy to prepare - just cut in half, season, and bake. They're an excellent source of iron, riboflavin and vitamins A and C, so they should be a welcome addition to your menu!

Serves 2-4

> 1 large acorn squash
> 2 Tablespoons olive oil
> 2 teaspoons maple syrup
> Salt and pepper

1. Preheat oven to 400 degrees.
2. Using a butcher knife, cut the acorn squash in half lengthwise, from stem to end. Scoop out the seeds and stringy threads from the center of each half.
3. Season the cavity of each squash with 1 tablespoon of olive oil, 1 teaspoon maple syrup, salt, and pepper. Place each half in a greased foil-lined pan, cut side down.
4. Bake in the oven for about 1 hour, until the squash is very soft and the tops are browned. Remove from oven and let cool a little before serving.

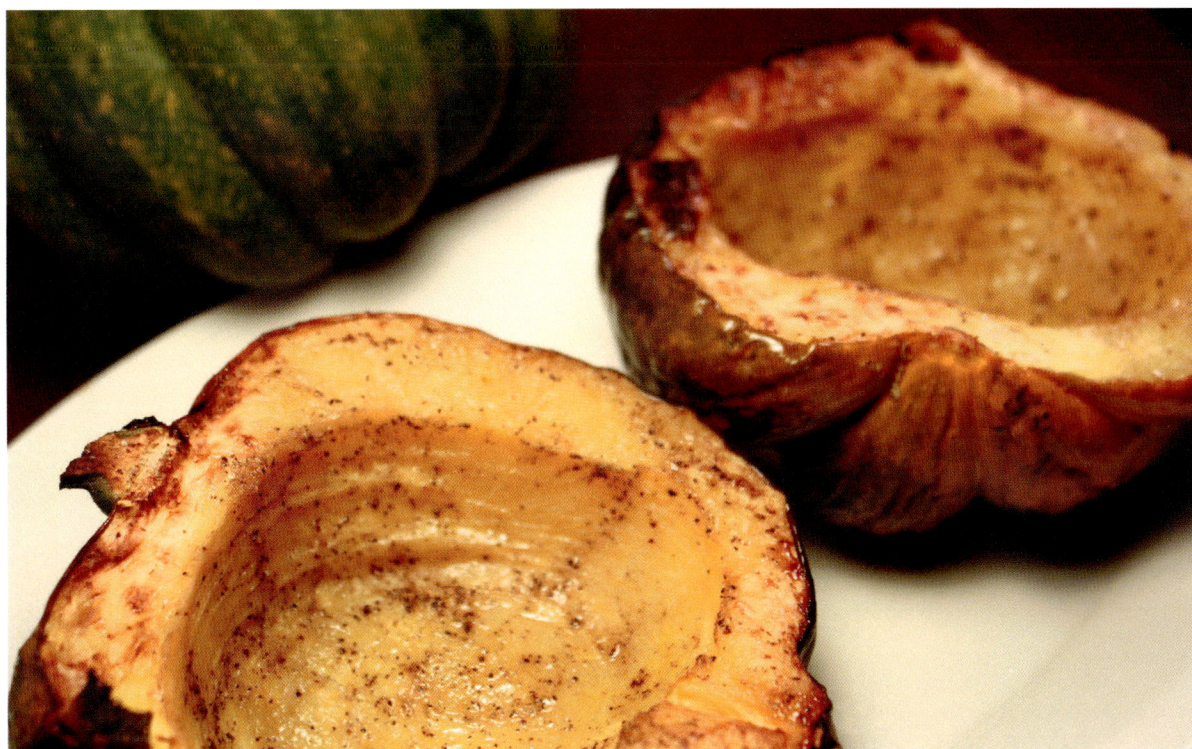

Snacks

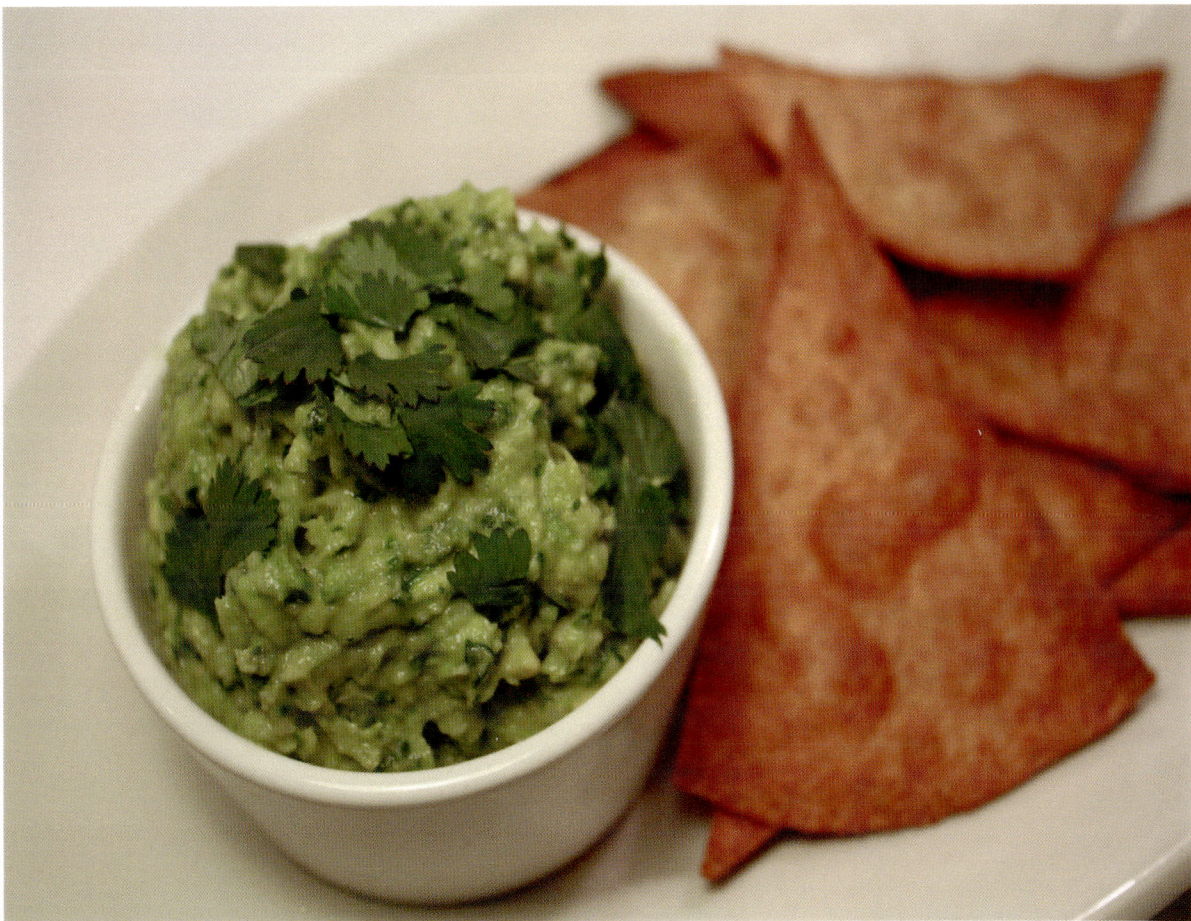

Chips & Guacamole

Chips & Guacamole

This recipe is the epitome of having your cake and eating it too - reinvented with a few smart modifications it's easy to enjoy your favorite foods during the Elimination Diet! The white beans in this guacamole add a creamy texture and an extra bit of hunger-busting fiber without compromising on taste!

Serves 2

Chips:

> Salt
> 2 brown rice tortillas, each sliced into 8 wedges (16 wedges total, like slicing pizza)
> Olive oil for frying

1. Pour olive oil into a cast iron skillet or wok to about one-half inch deep and heat on medium-high. Meanwhile, lay two paper towels on a plate for draining.
2. When the oil is hot (but not yet smoking), use tongs to individually place as many wedges as will easily fit into the skillet. Turn the wedges after 2 minutes to fry the other side, then fry for 2-3 minutes more until they are golden and slightly crisp (they'll get even crispier as they cool down).
3. Use tongs to remove the wedges and set on paper towels.
   Salt both sides immediately.
4. Continue with the remaining wedges, adding more oil to the skillet as needed.
5. Allow wedges to cool completely, which will ensure an extra crispy texture.

Tip: Olive oil has a much lower smoking point than vegetable oil, so use a lower heat and be careful when frying with olive oil - you certainly don't want to burn the tortillas or yourself!

Guacamole:

> 1 cup cooked white beans (cannellini or navy)
> 2 Tablespoons olive oil
> 4 large cloves garlic, minced
> 1 cup cilantro leaves and upper stems, roughly chopped
> 2 to 4 teaspoons ground cumin
> 1/2 teaspoon salt, or to taste
> 1 cup white or red onion, chopped and divided
> 3 medium ripe avocados, halved and pitted

1. In a blender, puree beans and olive oil until smooth. Transfer to a medium bowl.
2. In the same blender, place garlic, cilantro, cumin, salt, and 1/2 cup of the onion; pulse until thick. Add to bowl with bean mixture.
3. Scoop avocado from peel into the bowl with the bean mixture; mash with a fork until the mixture is blended but still chunky. Stir in the remaining 1/2 cup of onion.
4. Serve with brown rice tortilla chips.

Crispy Kale Chips

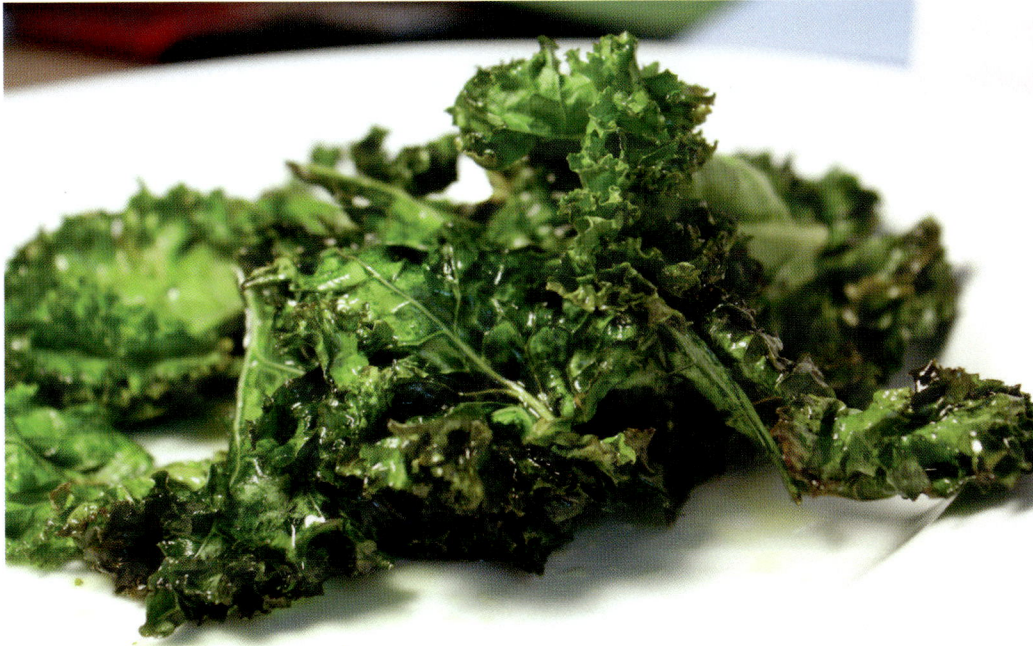

It's tempting to simply call these a substitute for potato chips, but don't be fooled - they're far superior!

Serves 4

> 1 bunch of lacinato or curly-leaf kale
> 1/4 cup olive oil
> Coarse sea salt

1. Preheat oven to 350 degrees.
2. Trim kale leaves by stripping each half of the leaves away from the tough center stems. Tear into large pieces.
3. Toss leaves in a large bowl with enough olive oil to lightly coat each leaf.
4. Spread leaves in a single layer on a baking sheet and roast for 5 minutes.
5. Turn the leaves over and roast another 5-10 minutes until kale begins to brown and is thin and brittle.
6. Remove from oven and sprinkle generously with sea salt.

Power Balls

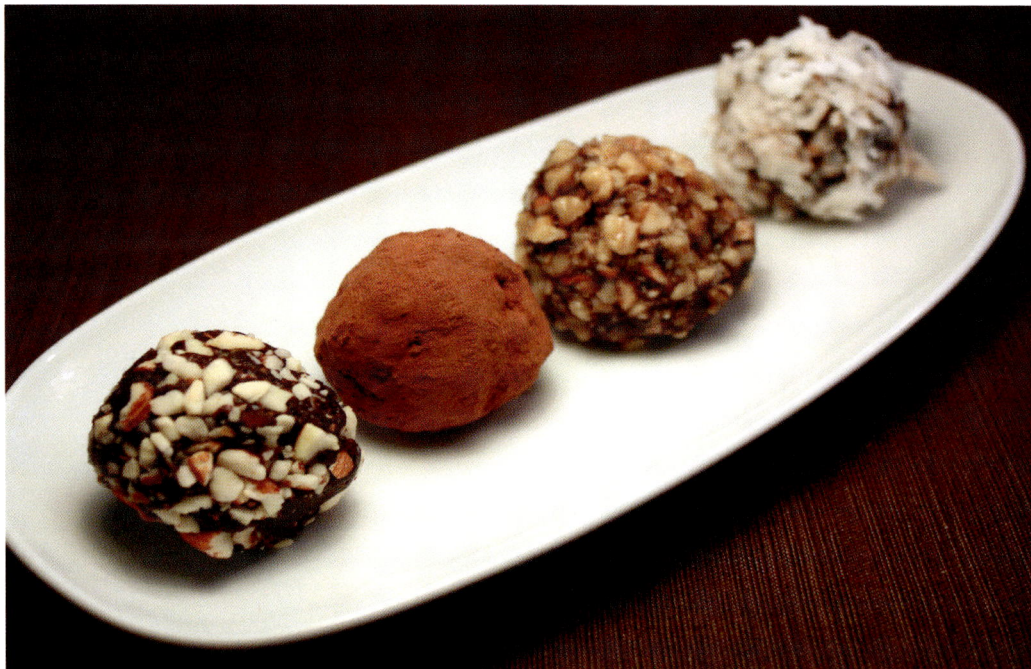

Just three steps to a great little raw cookie! These are fantastic to keep on hand for a quick pick-me-up or to satisfy a munchy craving.

Makes 8 balls

> 1 cup chopped dates
> 3/4 cup raw walnuts, almonds, or
>   pecans
> 1/4 cup carob powder
> Toppings: toasted coconut, finely chopped nuts, or additional carob powder

1. Place toppings in separate, small bowls.
2. Process the first three ingredients in a blender or food processor until sticky.
3. Shape into balls and roll through the toppings, as desired. Immediately put the balls in the fridge for 1/2 hour to firm up.

Hummus

Creamy, rich, and filling...what's not to love about hummus? Serve with sliced veggies and rice crackers for an easy snack and don't forget about presentation - hummus looks bland, so I like to dish it up in a colorful bowl and sprinkle it with parsley before serving.

Makes 2 cups, about 3-6 servings

> 1/2 cup onion, roughly chopped (about 1/4 large onion)
> 4 large cloves garlic, peeled and chopped
> 1 Tablespoon plus 1/4 cup olive oil, plus extra for drizzling
> 1 can garbanzo beans, undrained
> 1/2 cup tahini (sesame paste) with some of its oil, optional
> Salt to taste
> 1 to 1-1/2 teaspoons ground cumin, plus extra for garnish
> Chopped fresh parsley for garnish

1. Sauté onion and garlic in approximately 1 tablespoon olive oil until lightly browned.
2. Add onion mixture, garbanzo beans and liquid, tahini paste, 1/4 cup olive oil, salt, and cumin in a blender. Puree until smooth. (May need to add water for preferred consistency).
3. Serve, drizzled with the extra olive oil and sprinkled with additional cumin and parsley.

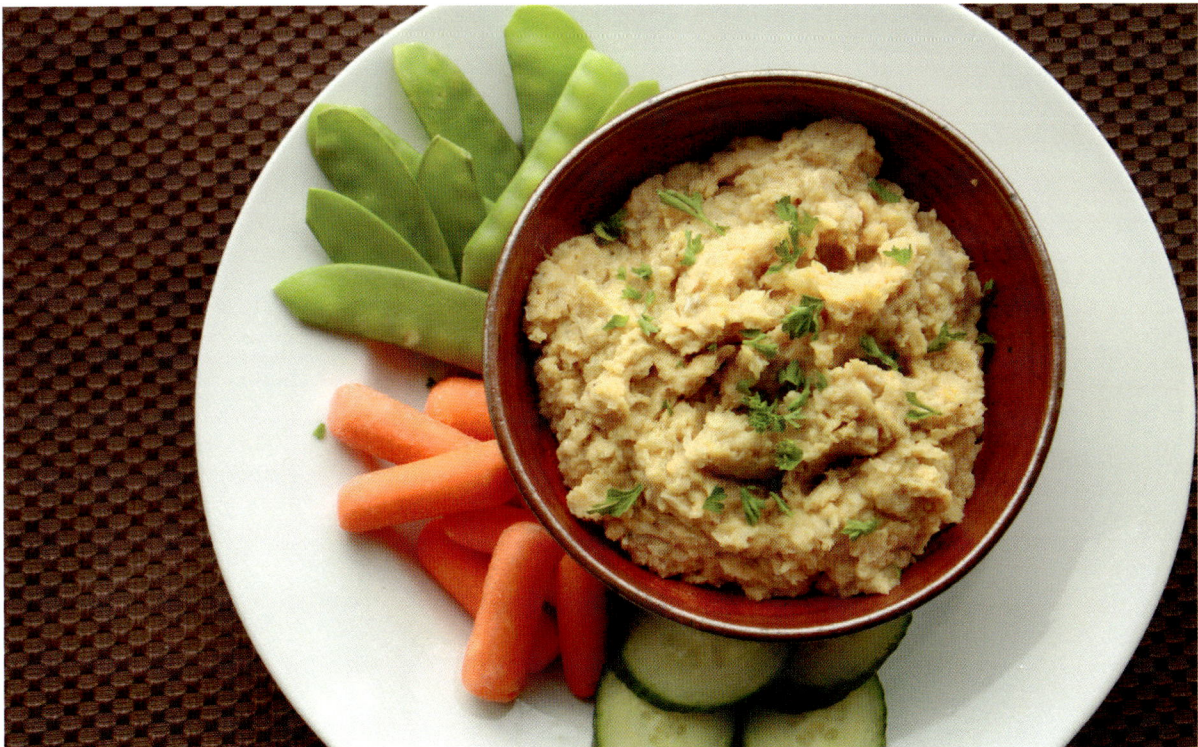

Roasted Sweet Potato Wedges

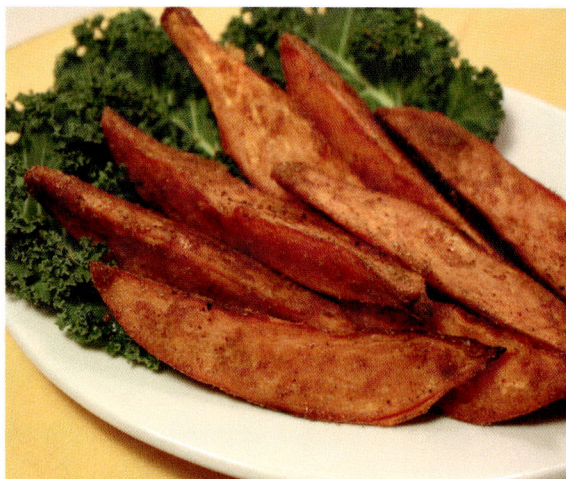

Craving French fries? These fries are sweet, salty, a bit spicy, and ultra nutritious - an unbeatable combination! Try to find potatoes that are more circular than long and thin, as it will be easier to cut the wedges into equal dimensions for even cooking. I eat these plain, but you might enjoy them dipped in spinach pesto or even guacamole.

Serves 4

Two 8-ounce sweet potatoes
1 teaspoon olive oil
1/2 teaspoon curry powder
1/4 teaspoon salt, plus extra to garnish
1/2 teaspoon cumin
1/8 teaspoon pepper
Spinach pesto, guacamole, or hummus to accompany, optional

1. Preheat oven to 425 degrees.
2. Cut each potato in half lengthwise into 6 wedges. Combine all ingredients in a bowl, toss to coat.
3. Place wedges in a single layer on a baking sheet, bake for 25 minutes or until very tender.
4. Sprinkle again with salt and serve with a dip (optional).

Peanut Dipping Sauce

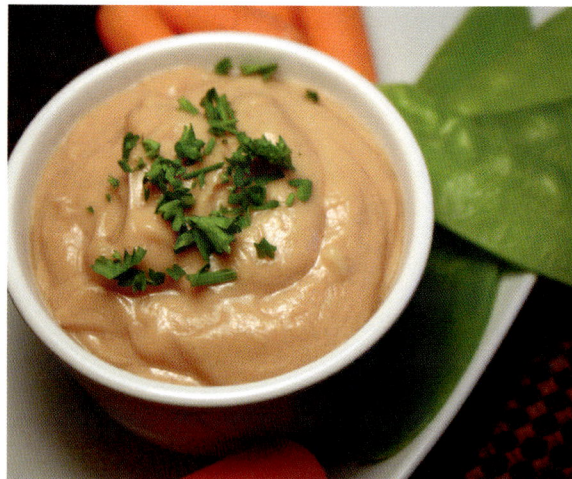

This simple blend can be used to accompany skewered chicken, sliced vegetables, or even watered down a bit and tossed with rice noodles. However you choose to serve it, you're sure to appreciate the easy preparation! Even better, it can be made a day or so in advance and kept covered in the fridge if you're short on time.

Makes about 1 cup

1/3 cup smooth peanut butter (not old fashioned or natural)
1 clove garlic
2 Tablespoons rice vinegar
2 Tablespoons sesame oil
2 teaspoons honey or brown rice syrup
1/3 cup coconut milk

1. Add all ingredients and blend gently until the mixture is smooth and transfer to a bowl.

Desserts

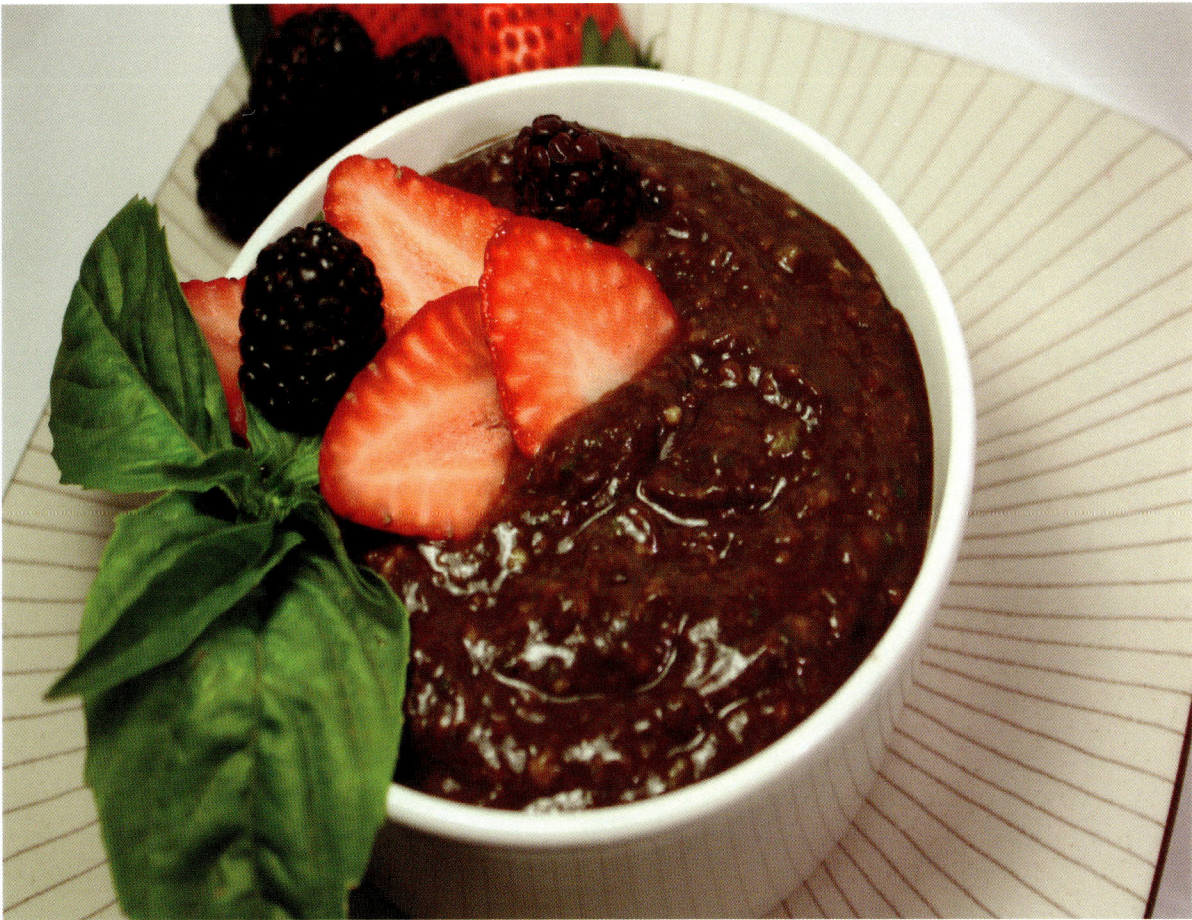

Carob Mousse

Carob Mousse

This delicious dessert really satisfies intense sugar cravings in the early days of the Elimination Diet. Carob is a healthy alternative to chocolate and cocoa - it's caffeine-free, tastes similar, contains little fat, and has triple the calcium! Look for it in the baking section of health food stores or online.

Adapted from *www.beautiful-vegan.com*

Serves 2

    1 large ripe avocado, pitted and peeled
    2 Tablespoons toasted carob powder
    1/4 to 1/3 cup honey or brown rice syrup, or Stevia to taste
    1/2 teaspoon salt (optional)
    2 teaspoon vanilla extract (or the scrapings from a vanilla bean pod)
    1/2 cup water or almond milk
    Blackberries or sliced strawberries to garnish

1. Combine the first six ingredients in a blender. Blend until smooth and thick. If necessary, add more water or milk to blend.
2. Dish into bowls and top with berries.

Tip: This mousse can do double-duty as a sorbet. Just place the mousse in the freezer overnight, then scoop out and enjoy!

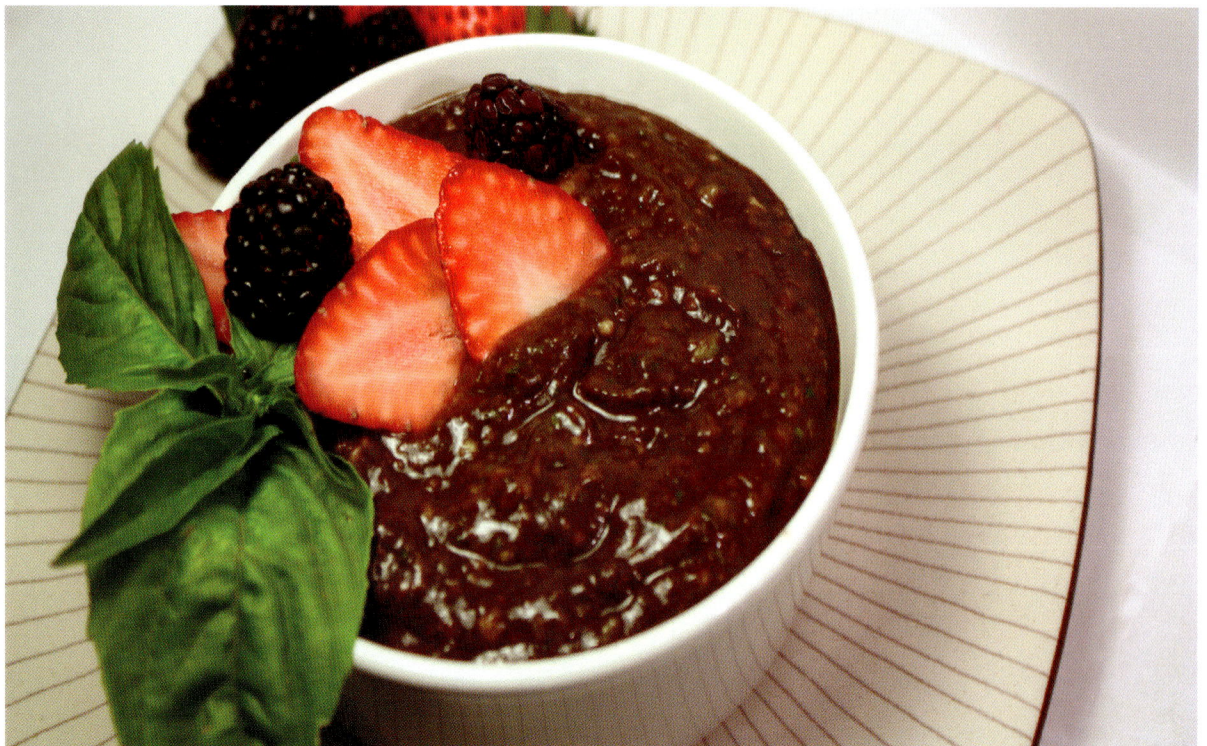

Pear Compote

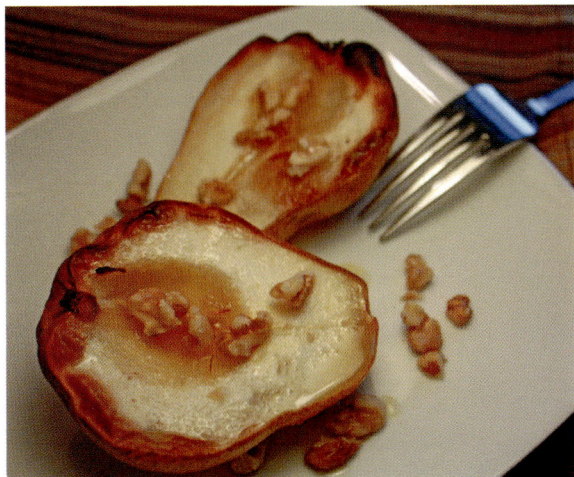

Here's a simple weeknight dessert that can bake while you're eating dinner. Pears keep decently in the refrigerator, so it's good to stock up when they're on sale - try doubling the recipe and serving the leftover pears for breakfast. Yum!

Serves 4

2 pears, halved and cored
4 teaspoons oil (walnut, olive, or
   coconut), plus more to grease pan
4 teaspoons honey or brown rice syrup
1/4 cup toasted walnuts
Cinnamon or nutmeg

1. Preheat oven to 350 degrees.
2. Place pears, cavity up, in a baking pan lightly greased with oil. Drizzle cut side and cavity with 1 teaspoon each of the oil and honey.
3. Cover pan and bake until very soft, about 30 minutes.
4. Sprinkle each pear with walnuts and a pinch of cinnamon or nutmeg. Serve warm.

Banana Ice Cream

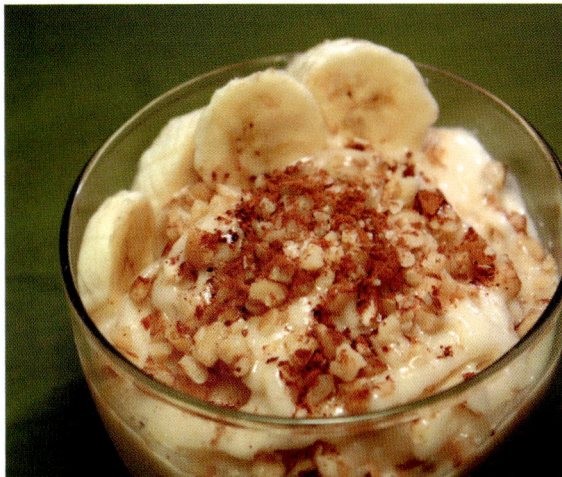

One of my favorite challenges is persuading newcomers to the Elimination Diet that there is a divine-tasting Elimination Diet-friendly equivalent for nearly every man-made concoction they crave. Nothing demonstrates this better than the following recipe, though I hesitate to call it a recipe because it's so darn simple. After trying it, be prepared to buy bananas in bulk!

Serves 1

1 banana, peeled and frozen in large
   chunks
3 Tablespoons almond milk
1-1/2 teaspoon vanilla
Toppings (optional): chopped walnuts
or pecans, carob nibs, chopped dates,
or shredded coconut

1. Add banana, almond milk, and vanilla into a blender. Blend on medium for several minutes until the mixture is thick.
2. Add toppings and serve immediately.

Tip: For chocolate-flavored ice cream, add 1 teaspoon carob powder to bananas and milk before blending.

Rice Crispy Crunchies

Remember the marshmallow-y rice crispy treat squares you devoured as a kid? Here's the Elimination Diet version! The batter is quite gooey and will stick to dry hands, so keep your hands constantly wet when forming the clusters - I like to leave a small bowl of water next to the blender so I don't have to run back and forth from the sink. These little clusters can be enjoyed at room temperature, but they soften and so should be stored in the fridge for a firmer crunch.

Makes 12 Crunchies

> 1/4 cup almond butter
> 3 Tablespoon carob powder
> 1 Tablespoon honey or brown rice syrup
> 2 teaspoons flax, walnut, or melted coconut oil
> 6 to 8 Tablespoons crispy brown rice cereal, plus 1/3 cup for rolling

1. Place the first four ingredients in a bowl and stir to combine until well mixed. Add 6-8 tablespoons of the rice cereal and stir gently to combine.
2. Put 1/3 cup rice cereal in a small bowl.
3. Wet hands thoroughly. Between palms of hands, shape and roll 1 tablespoon of batter into a tight ball. Roll the ball in the bowl of rice cereal to cover.
4. Immediately put the Crunchies in the fridge for 1/2 hour to firm up.

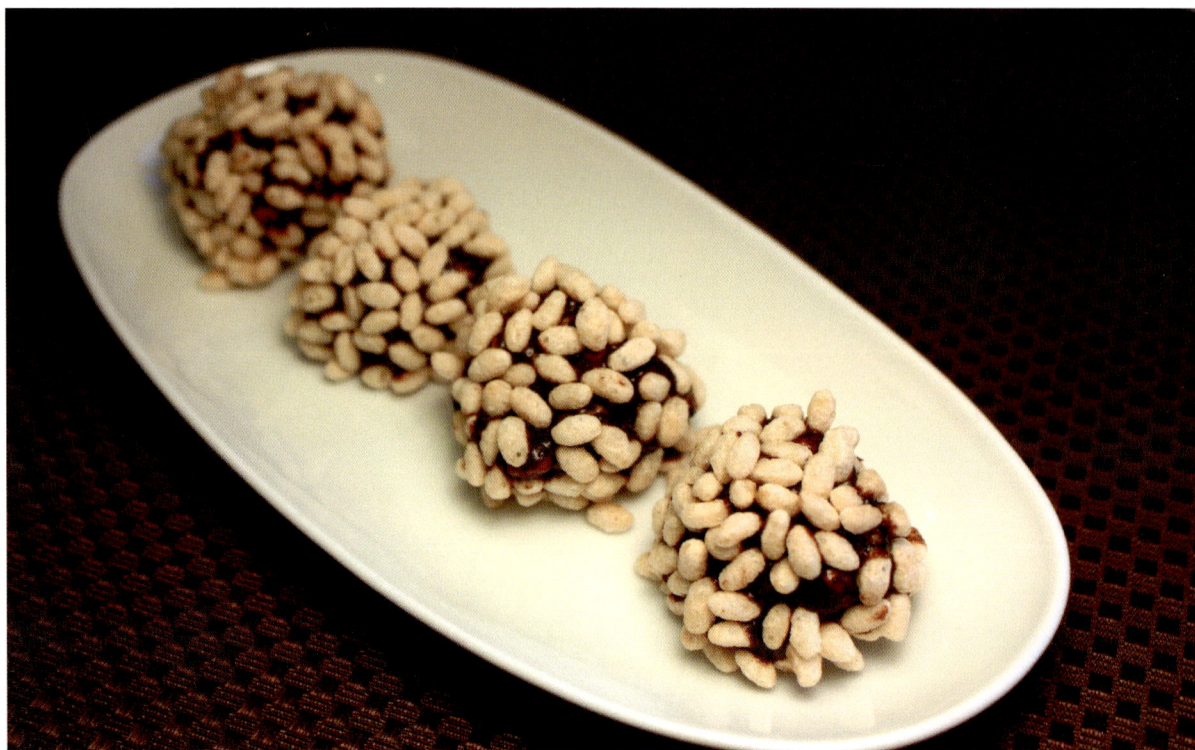

Autumn Spice Latte

For the coffee zealots among you (and you know who you are!), the true sign that fall has arrived is the annual reappearance of Starbucks' Pumpkin Spice Latte. There's no need to totally miss out on this cult ritual - this spicy, sweet, and creamy blend is a healthy replica that won't disappoint.

Inspired by *www.healthfulpursuit.com*

Serves 1

1 cup almond milk
1/2 cup mashed sweet potato or canned pumpkin
1/2 banana
1 Tablespoon maple syrup
1/2 teaspoon vanilla extract
1/2 to 1 teaspoon pumpkin pie spice, to taste
Nutmeg or cinnamon

1. Combine all ingredients except nutmeg in a blender.
2. Blend until smooth.
3. Pour into a large mug and sprinkle with nutmeg or cinnamon.

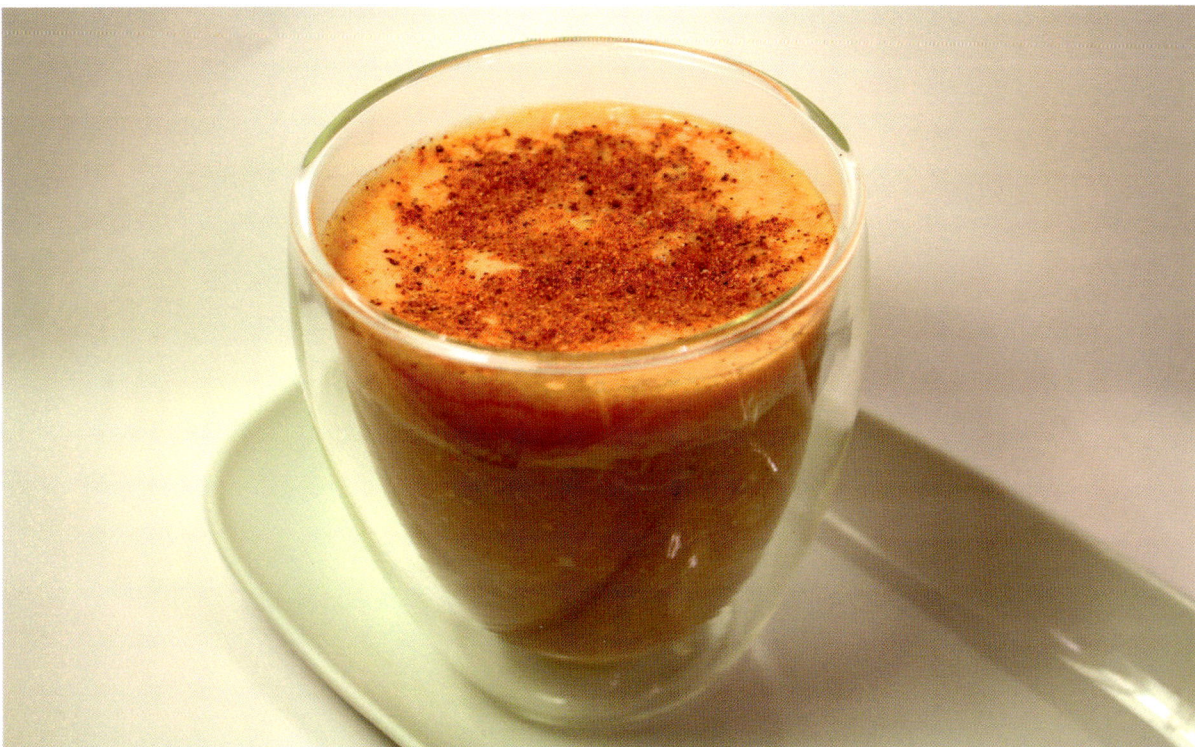

Challenge Phase

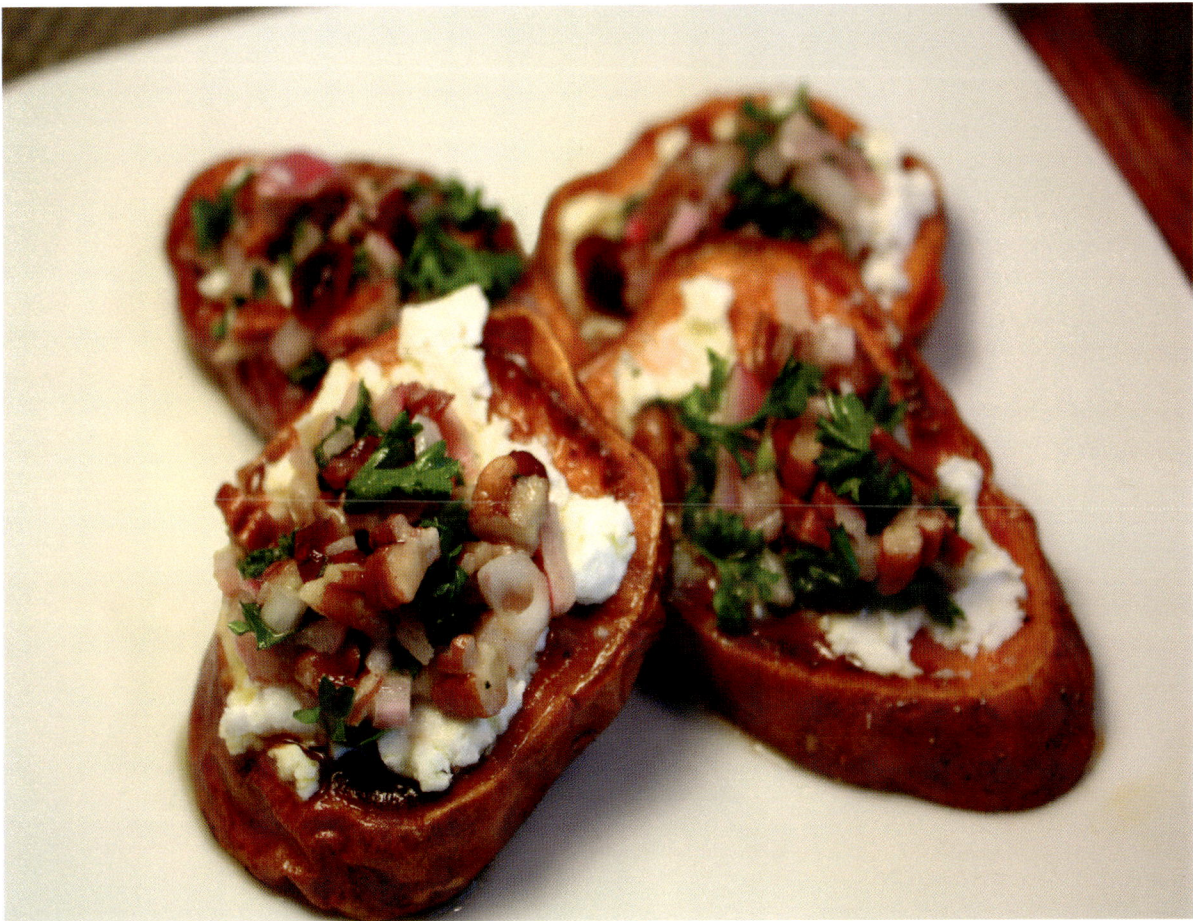

Sweet Potato & Goat Cheese Bruschetta

Lavender Lemonade

I was first introduced to this refreshing drink at a picturesque lavender farm in the San Juan Islands where my family frequently visited when I was a little girl. It made such a big impression that I'm still enjoying it 20 years later! You might want to add a bit more honey or maple syrup depending on your taste, but I personally feel that the tart lemons allow the lavender essence to really shine.

Serves 4

2 cups water
2 Tablespoons lavender flower buds
3 lemons
1 quart water
1/4 cup honey or maple syrup to taste
Fresh lavender flower spikes for garnish, optional

1. Bring 2 cups of water to a boil.
2. Add lavender, cover the pan, and let it steep for about 30 minutes.
3. Strain and reserve the liquid. (This is the lavender extract that you will use later.)
4. Roll the lemons on a hard surface to help release the juices. Cut and squeeze them to create about 1/2 cup of juice, straining out the seeds.
5. To one quart of water, add lemon juice, honey, and 2 cups of the lavender extract. Stir well to dissolve.
6. Chill, serve over ice. Garnish with lavender spikes.

Tip: If you're in a crafty mood and want to elevate this beverage to "special guest" status, you can make your own lavender ice to add with the lemonade. Just drop a few lavender flowers in the ice cube tray squares before freezing the water. Beautiful!

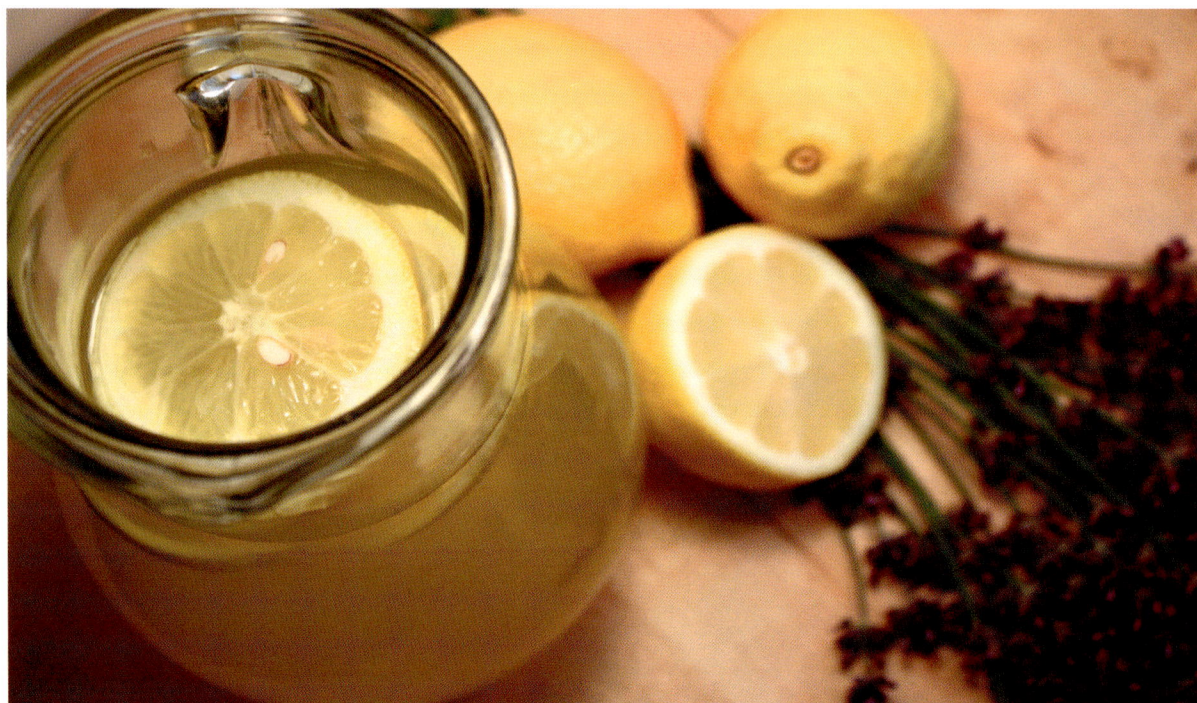

Coconut Lime Chicken

This is one of the dishes that I missed the most during the Elimination Phase of the Elimination Diet. Hopefully that's enough of an endorsement to convince you to try it! Alongside a simple green salad to counter the sweetness of the coconut, this is an indulgent dish that can be prepared in a flash for week-night dinners!

Adapted from *www.realsimple.com*

Serves 4

4 medium boneless, skinless chicken breasts
Salt and pepper
1 Tablespoon olive oil or coconut oil
2 cloves garlic, chopped
One 14-ounce can light coconut milk
Shredded zest and juice of 1 large lime
1 Tablespoon Thai fish sauce, optional
2 Tablespoons chopped cilantro
3 cups cooked brown rice

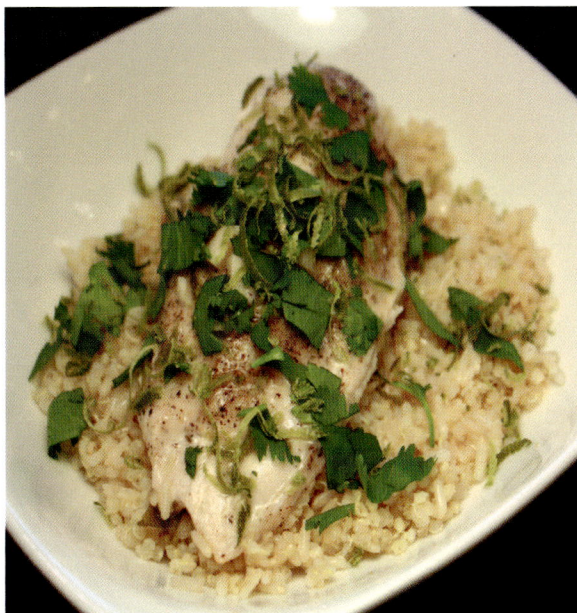

1. Pound the chicken with a rolling pin to uniform thickness. Season both sides with salt and pepper.
2. Heat the oil and garlic in a large skillet over medium-high heat until the garlic softens (but do not let the garlic burn). Add the chicken breasts and cook until golden, 4-5 minutes per side.
3. Add the coconut milk, lime zest, and lime juice. Stir, cover, and reduce heat to medium-low. Cook 3 minutes longer until the chicken is tender.
4. Remove chicken to a platter and keep warm. Increase heat to high and boil the sauce until thickened, 4-5 minutes.
5. Whisk in the Thai fish sauce (if using) and pour the sauce over the chicken. Sprinkle with cilantro, and serve over brown rice.

Tip: Per the notes in the Curried Vegetable Soup recipe (see the Soups section), it's much cheaper to make your own "light" coconut milk from regular canned coconut milk than to buy a can of light milk, but the light canned version is also available in most grocery stores too if you are short on time or motivation.

Grapefruit Brulee

Breakfast? Dessert? I can't ever make my mind up as to when this simple little dish should be served. With a unique combination of sweet and tart flavors, grapefruit can easily be enjoyed in a range of sweet to savory dishes. Not to mention that it's one of the few things to look forward to in the produce aisle during the harsh winter season!

Serves 2

1 large grapefruit, halved
2 Tablespoons honey or maple syrup
1/4 teaspoon nutmeg
1/4 teaspoon cinnamon, plus more to serve

1. Preheat broiler with rack set 4-5 inches from heat.
2. Using a small paring knife, loosen fruit segments from the pith and membranes.
3. Drizzle 1 tablespoon honey over each grapefruit half and sprinkle with nutmeg and cinnamon.
4. Broil on a lined baking sheet until the tops are moderately browned and bubbling, about 5-6 minutes.
5. Garnish with more cinnamon and serve.

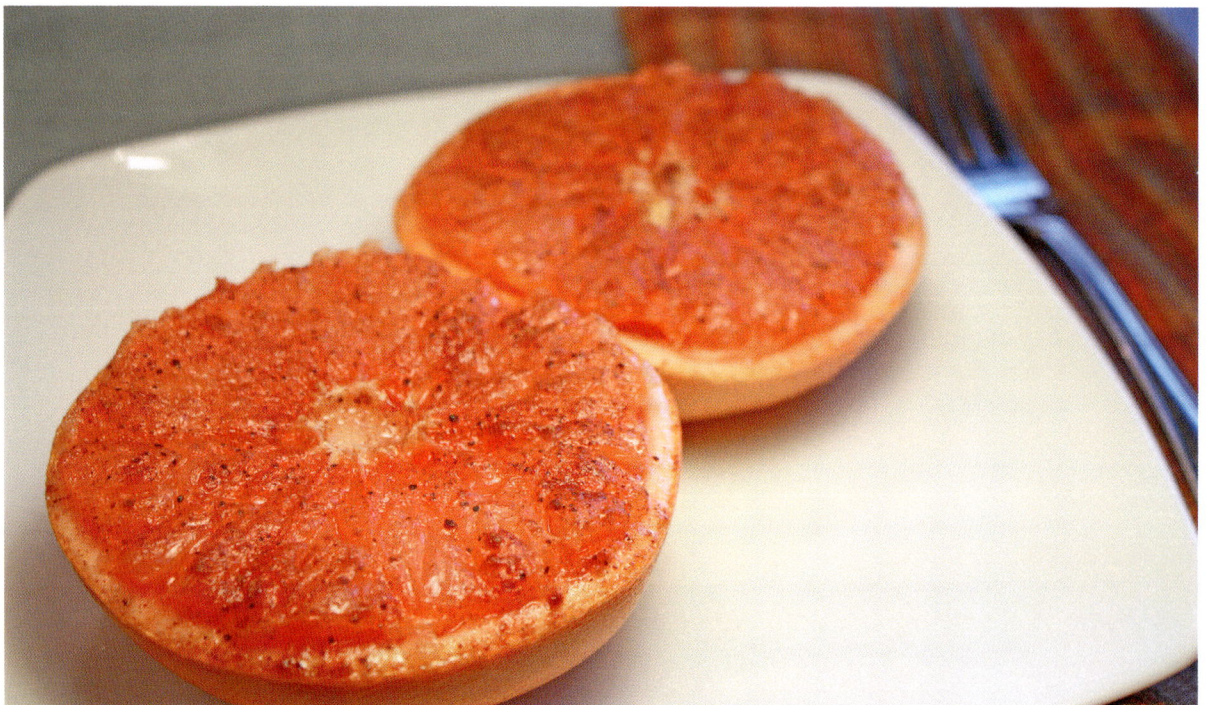

Warm Chicken Citrus Salad

A few summers ago, like many novice gardeners, I got carried away planting too many lettuce starts.
They looked so small - little did I know how big they would get as the days grew longer and warmer! In an effort to help me exploit the astronomical surplus of leaves, a friend traded this recipe in exchange for a bag of lettuce - I definitely got the better end of the deal!

Serves 4

- 2 medium oranges, peeled
- 6 cups torn romaine lettuce
- 1/2 of a small red onion, halved and thinly sliced
- 1/3 cup slivered or sliced almonds, toasted
- 1 cup sliced cucumbers
- 1 pound skinless, boneless chicken breast cut into thin bite-size strips
- Salt and pepper
- 2 Tablespoons olive oil
- 1 large avocado, diced or sliced
- 1/3 cup orange juice
- 1 Tablespoon red wine vinegar
- 1 teaspoon spicy mustard
- Coarsely ground black pepper

1. Cut oranges into 1/4-inch slices; quarter each orange slice. In a large salad bowl toss together orange chunks, lettuce, onion, almonds, and cucumber. Set aside mixture.
2. Season chicken with salt and black pepper. In a large skillet heat 1 tablespoon oil to medium high, then add chicken and sauté for 4 to 5 minutes or until no longer pink. Remove skillet from heat. Toss chicken with mixture in salad bowl. Divide salad among 4 dinner plates. Sprinkle avocado on top of the salads.
3. Stir orange juice and vinegar into the hot skillet, scraping up any brown bits in the skillet. Whisk in remaining 1 tablespoon of olive oil and the mustard, and cook over medium-high heat just until bubbles begin to appear.
4. Pour the warm dressing over salads and season to taste with coarsely ground black pepper to serve.

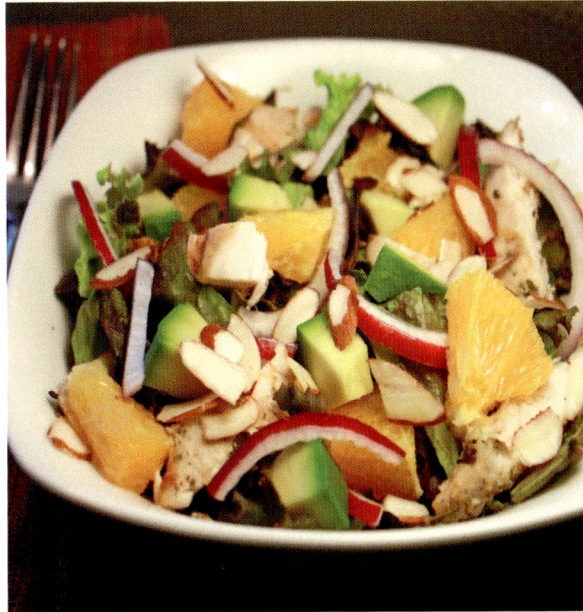

Roasted Corn on the Cob

Once you try this version of corn on the cob, you might never want it prepared any other way! Friends for whom I've made this recipe now understand why I get so excited when fresh corn makes its annual autumnal debut at the neighborhood Farmers' Market.

Serves 4

> 4 ears corn with husks left on
> Salt and pepper

1. Preheat oven to 350 degrees. Gently rinse and dry ears, keeping husks on.
2. Place ears directly on middle rack of heated oven and bake for 30 minutes.
3. Let ears cool slightly, then pull back husks. Season with salt and pepper to serve.

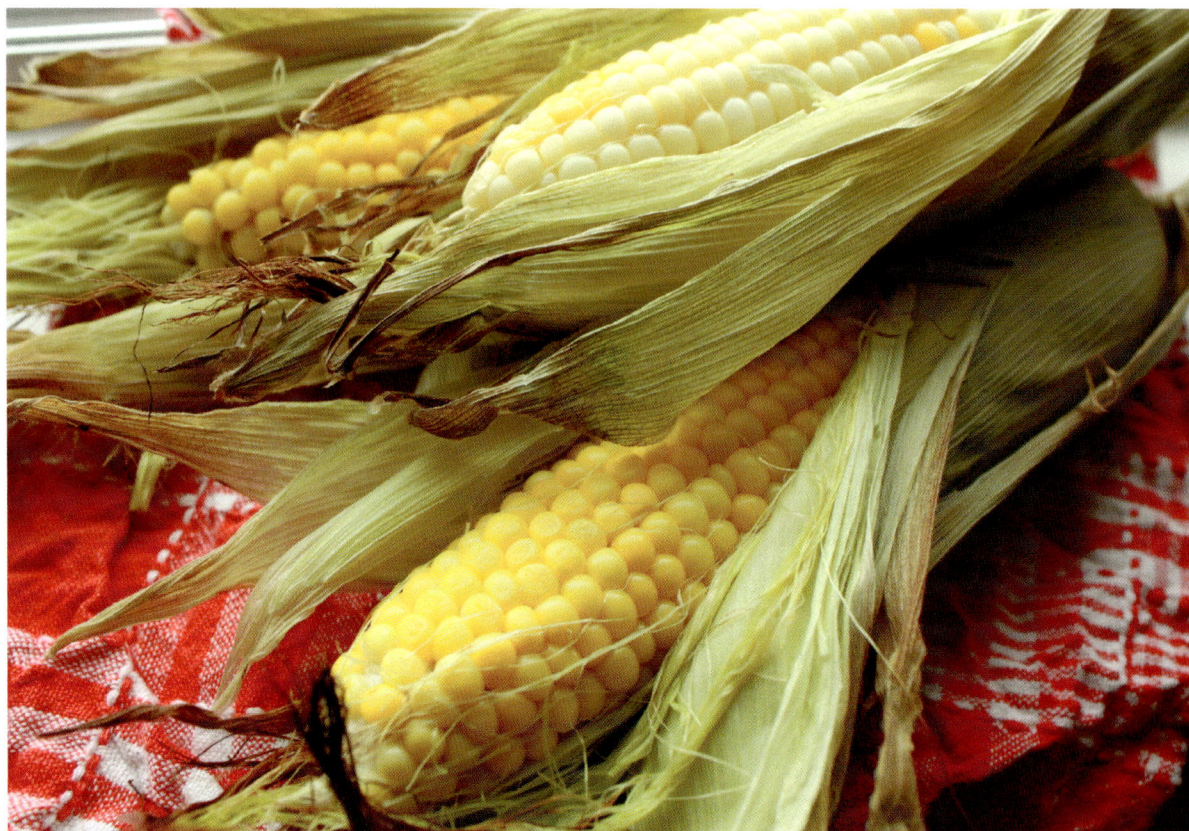

Sweet Potato & Goat Cheese Bruschetta

You'll have an easy time of the Elimination Diet if you can invent easy substitutes for your favorite foods. Here, sweet potatoes and a nut salsa do a brilliant and colorful imitation of the more traditional bruschetta with bread and tomatoes. If you're planning to serve this dish again as leftovers, don't dress all the potato rounds at once - keep everything separate to ensure it is bright and fresh for later!

Inspired by *www.smittenkitchen.com*

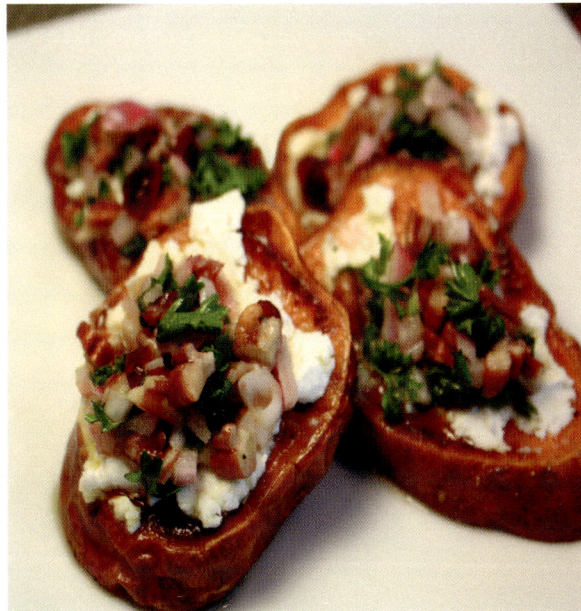

Serves 4

- 2 Tablespoons plus 1/4 cup olive oil
- 3 pounds sweet potato, unpeeled and cut in 1/2-inch coins
- Salt and pepper
- 1/2 cup toasted and cooled pecan halves, chopped
- 2 small shallots, minced
- 1/4 cup Italian parsley, chopped
- 2 Tablespoons dried cranberries, minced
- 4 ounces goat cheese
- 4 teaspoons red wine vinegar
- 1 teaspoon smooth mustard

1. Preheat oven to 450 degrees. Coat a large baking sheet with 2 tablespoons olive oil. Lay sweet potatoes in one layer on the oiled sheet. Sprinkle with salt and pepper.
2. Roast, without disturbing, for 15-20 minutes until the underside is somewhat dark and a bit puffy. Flip and sprinkle them again with additional salt and pepper and return the pan to the oven for another 10 minutes or so, until the new undersides are also cooked.
3. Meanwhile, combine the pecans, shallots, parsley, and cranberries. If using firm goat cheese, crumble and stir it into the mixture. If the goat cheese is softer, set it aside to be spread on top of the potato rounds.
4. Prepare the dressing: in a small dish, whisk together 1/4 cup olive oil, red wine vinegar, and mustard. Pour half of this mixture over the topping and gently mix.
5. Transfer potato rounds to a serving platter. (If using soft goat cheese, spread it evenly across each of the potato rounds). Scoop a spoonful of the mixture over each round. Pour remaining salad dressing over top. Serve immediately.

Yogurt Medley

There's just something magical about this deceptively simple concoction of pantry staples...tart, sweet, crunchy, and creamy all at the same time. My advice? Double the recipe because you're going to want to devour the leftovers for lunch.

Serves 2

> 1 large apple, cored, quartered, and coarsely grated
> 1-1/2 cups plain yogurt
> 1/4 cup dates
> 2 Tablespoons honey or maple syrup
> 1/4 cup sliced almonds
> Cinnamon to garnish

1. In a small mixing bowl, combine apple, yogurt, dates, and honey; divide between two serving bowls.
2. Sprinkle with almonds and cinnamon, if using, and serve immediately.

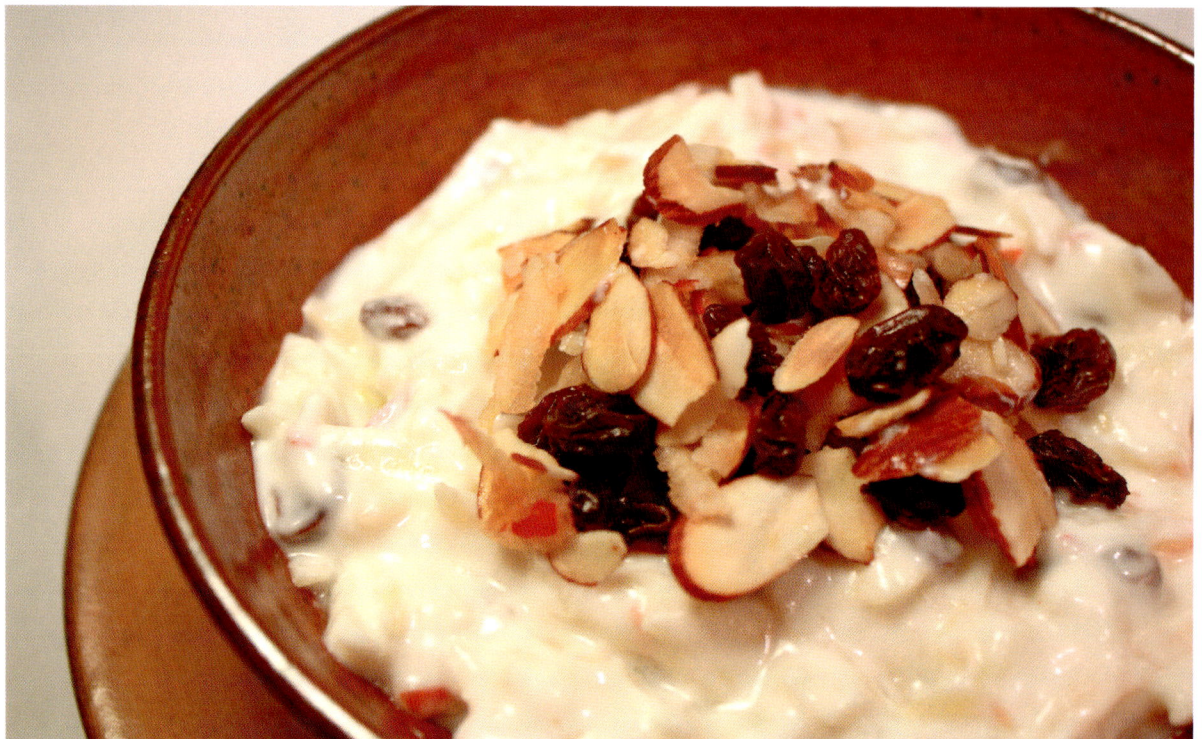

Eggs Anemone

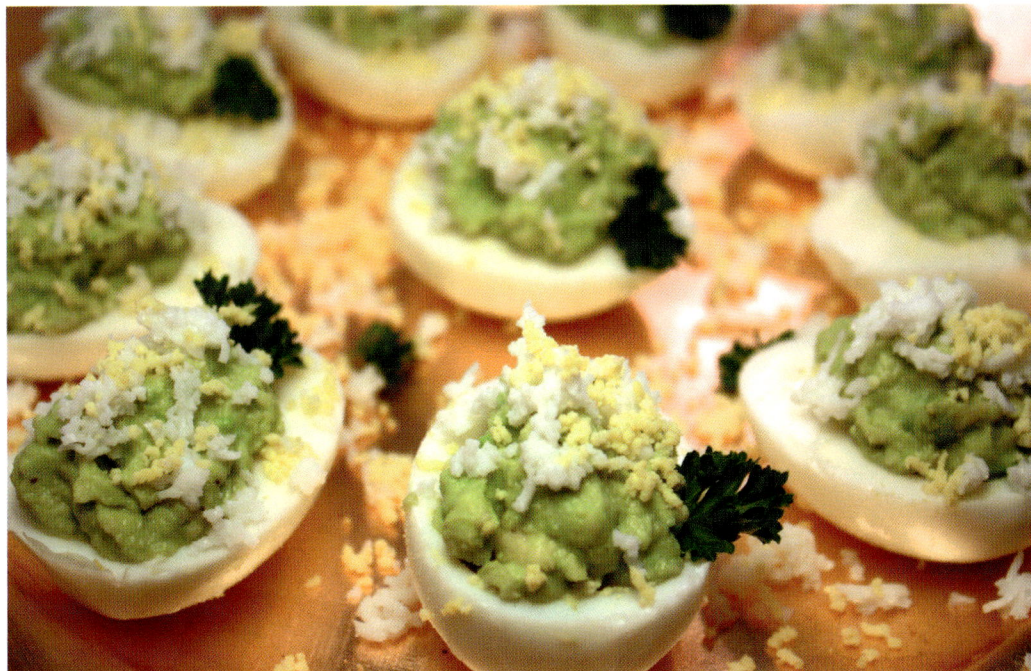

Anemone describes the fine yellow and white grated eggs in this dish, which resemble the flower of the same name. Be ready to serve this fun yet sophisticated appetizer soon after preparing, as avocado tends to brown quickly once exposed to air.

Inspired by Joanna Farrow's *Four Ingredients Cookbook*

Makes 10

> 6 eggs, hard-boiled and peeled
> 1 large ripe avocado halved and pitted
> 1 small clove garlic, crushed
> 1 Tablespoon olive oil
> Salt and pepper
> Basil or parsley leaves to garnish, optional

1. Reserve one of the eggs and halve the remaining five eggs. Carefully remove the yolks with a teaspoon. Blend the yolks with the avocados, garlic and oil, adding salt and pepper to taste.
2. Spoon or pipe the avocado mixture evenly into the halved egg whites.
3. Sieve the remaining egg whites and sprinkle over the filled eggs. Sieve the yolks and sprinkle on top.
4. Arrange the filled eggs on a plate and sprinkle with more black pepper and basil leaves, if using.

Tip: If you like the more formal look of piped filling but don't have piping bags and nozzles, simply spoon the mixture into a ziplock bag and cut a small hole in the bottom corner of one side. Pipe the material out of that small hole.

Apple Pie Crockpot Oatmeal

If you haven't yet discovered the joys of owning a slow cooker, this single recipe might be justification enough to run out and purchase one immediately. That is, unless you don't like apple pie or its wonderful aroma wafting throughout the house overnight as it cooks!

Serves 6

2 Tablespoons walnut or coconut oil
2 cups steel cut oats
1/4 cup flax seeds (optional)
1 to 2 Tablespoons vanilla
1 to 2 Tablespoons cinnamon
1 large apple, cored and chopped
1/2 cup chopped dates (optional)
1 cup chopped walnuts
8 cups water or almond milk (or a combination)
2 bananas, sliced (optional)
Maple syrup, to taste
Additional almond milk, if desired

1. Coat the inside of a 6-quart slow cooker with the oil.
2. Add oats, flax seeds, vanilla, cinnamon, apple, dates, and walnuts then stir to mix.
3. Add water or almond milk, cover, and cook on low for 7-8 hours.
4. Stir in banana slices and serve drizzled with maple syrup and topped with additional almond milk.

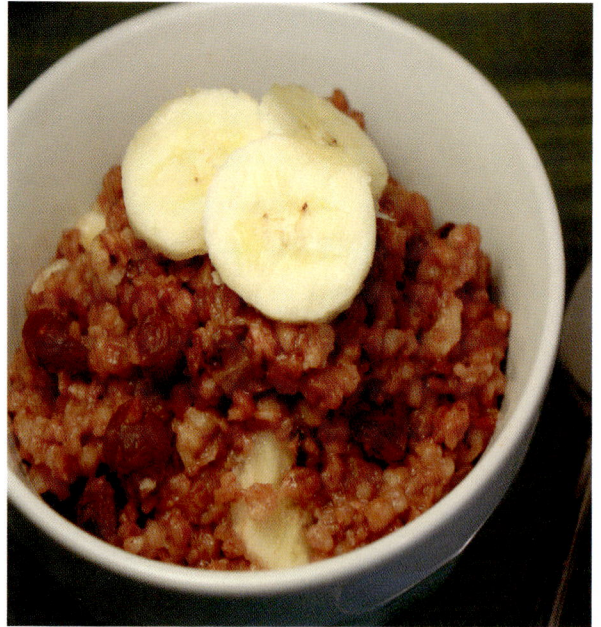

Fun Fact: Oats are safe for most people who are gluten-intolerant, but there is a small segment of gluten-intolerant people who also have a hard time with oats. Some researchers believe that reactions come from cross contamination in the oats (which can be processed in facilities that also process other grains), while others claim that there is a specific sensitivity to oats. Either way, it's enough of a debate that oats are included as part of the Elimination Diet regimen.

Rye & Seed Crackers

This seedy, crunchy cracker is quite versatile and can be modified to include any seeds or herbs that you enjoy - caraway, chia, flax, basil, garlic salt, etc.

Serves 4-8

1 cup rye flour
1 cup garbanzo bean flour, plus extra for rolling
Salt
1/8 teaspoon baking soda
1/4 cup olive oil
1/2 cup water
1 Tablespoon fennel seeds
1 Tablespoon sesame seeds
1 Tablespoon poppy seeds

1. Preheat oven to 375 degrees.
2. Mix all ingredients together. Add more water if necessary to make a sticky ball.
3. Roll out very thinly on a large floured sheet of wax paper.
4. Cut dough into desired shapes.
5. Transfer wax paper with cut dough directly onto a cookie sheet and bake for about 30 minutes.

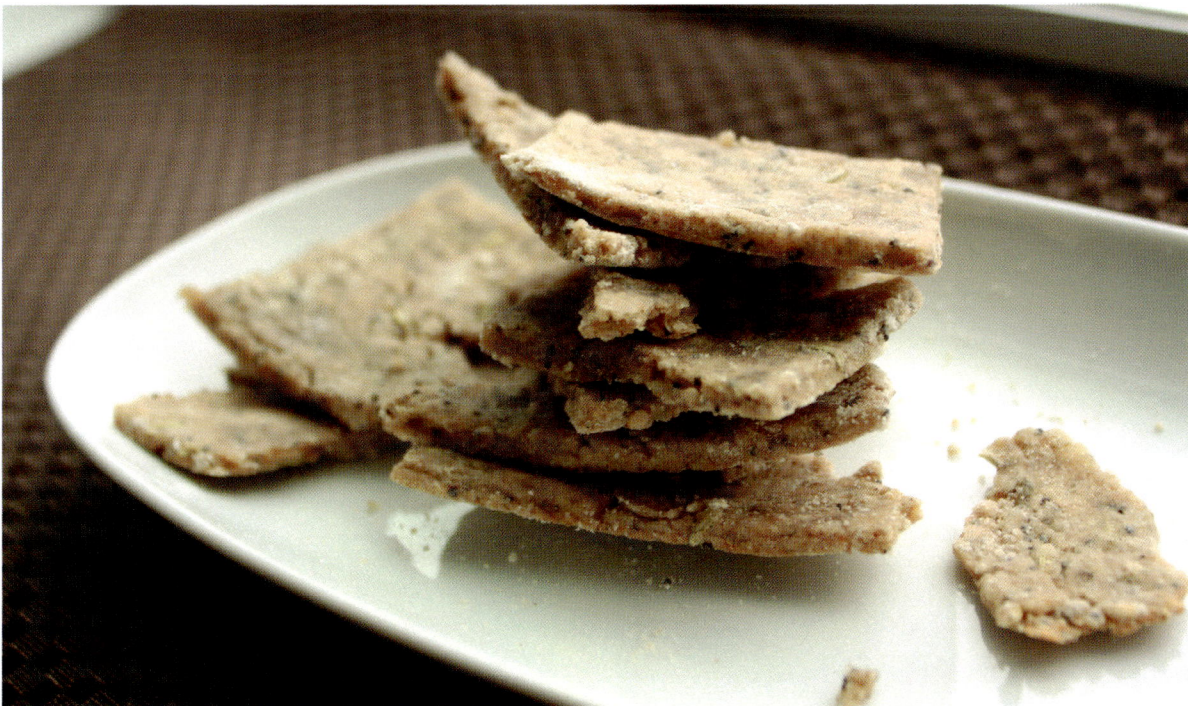

Barley & Rice Pilaf

I know this looks too simple to actually taste good, but it really does! The barley adds just a hint of nuttiness that makes this side dish anything but bland. This batch will leave you with plenty of leftovers, so it's a good thing that this recipe freezes well!

Serves 8-10

> 1 cup onion, chopped
> 1 Tablespoon olive oil
> 2 cups short-grain brown rice
> 1/2 cup pearl barley
> 3-1/2 cups chicken stock or water
> 1/2 cup chopped almonds (optional)

1. Sauté onion in a large pot with the olive oil.
2. Add the rice, barley, and stock. Bring to a boil.
3. Reduce heat to low and cover. Cook for 40-50 minutes.
4. Remove from heat and let stand, covered, for 10-15 minutes. Toss with almonds.

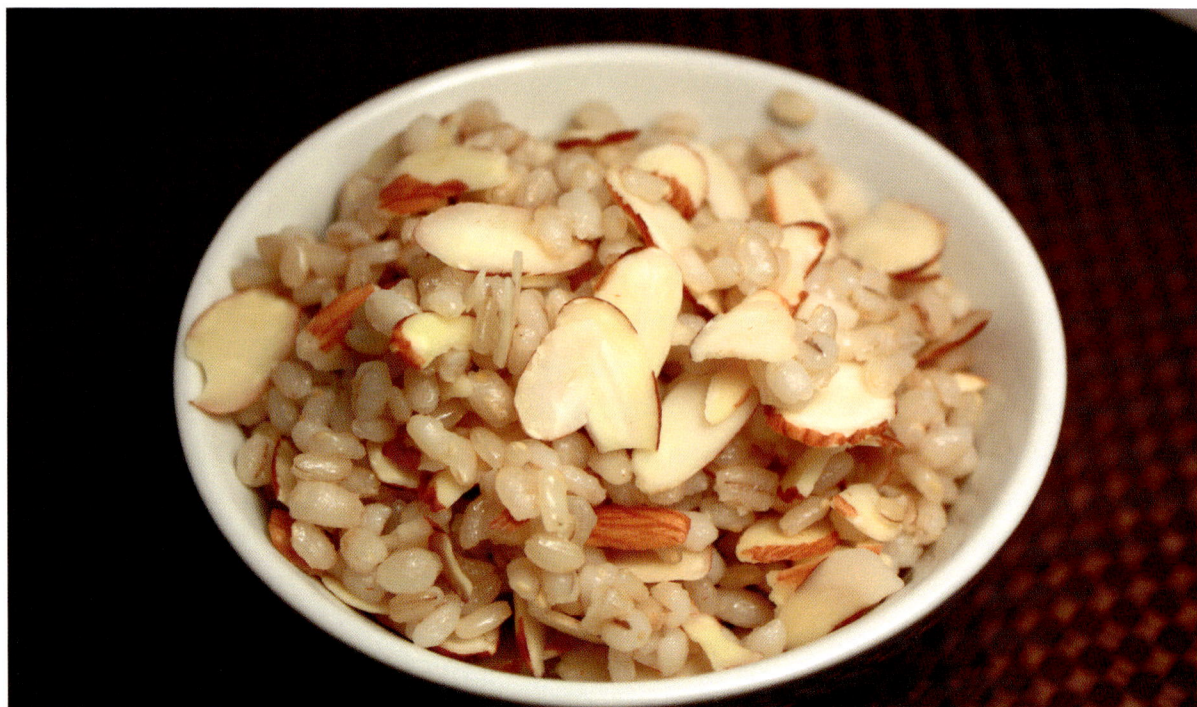

Chicken & Bulgur Pilaf

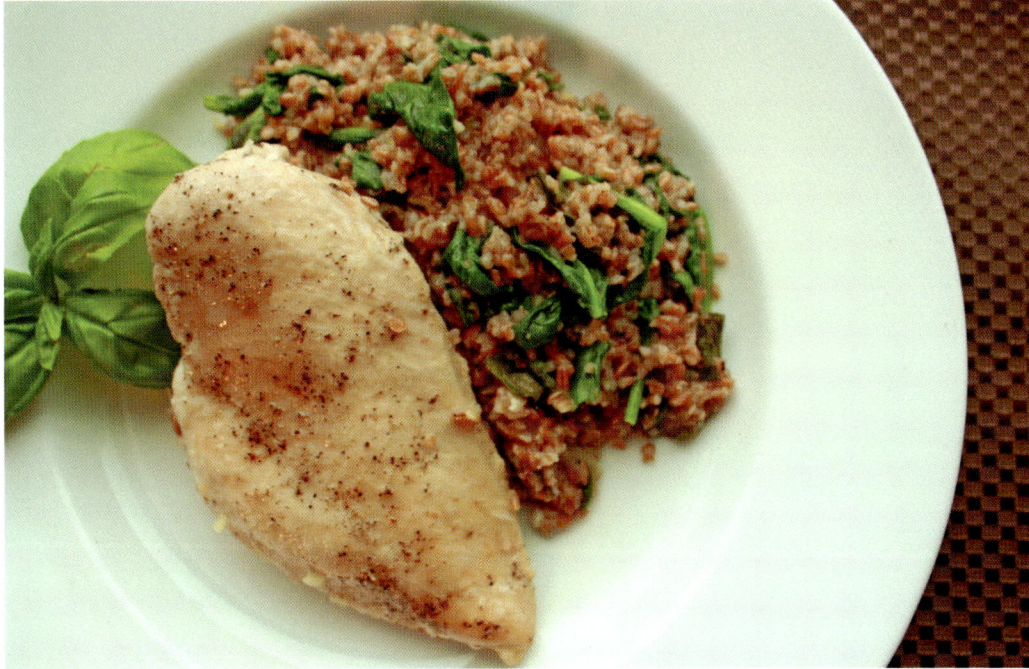

Bulgur, a Middle Eastern staple, is what's left after wheat berry kernels have been steamed, dried, and crushed. This nutty grain is a wonderful substitute for rice - it's quick to prepare, high in fiber, and loaded with B vitamins. You might need to head to the health food store or bulk bins to find it, as it's not yet the widely-popular grain it should be!

Inspired by *www.realsimple.com*

Serves 4

> 1 Tablespoon olive oil
> Four 6-ounce boneless, skinless chicken breasts
> Salt and pepper to taste
> 3 cups chicken or vegetable broth
> 1-1/2 cups medium-grain bulgur
> 2 cloves garlic, chopped
> 1 bunch spinach (about 3 cups), thick stems removed and coarsely chopped
> 1/2 cup fresh basil leaves, torn

1. Heat the olive oil in a large skillet over medium-high heat. Season the chicken with salt and pepper and cook until golden, 3 to 4 minutes per side. Transfer to a plate.
2. Add broth, bulgur, garlic, salt, and pepper to the skillet and bring to a boil.
3. Nestle the chicken in the bulgur, reduce heat to low, cover, and simmer until the bulgur is tender and the chicken is cooked through, 15 to 17 minutes.
4. Transfer the chicken to plates. Add the spinach and basil to the bulgur, stir until slightly wilted, and serve with the chicken.

Sweet Potato Chicken Quesadillas

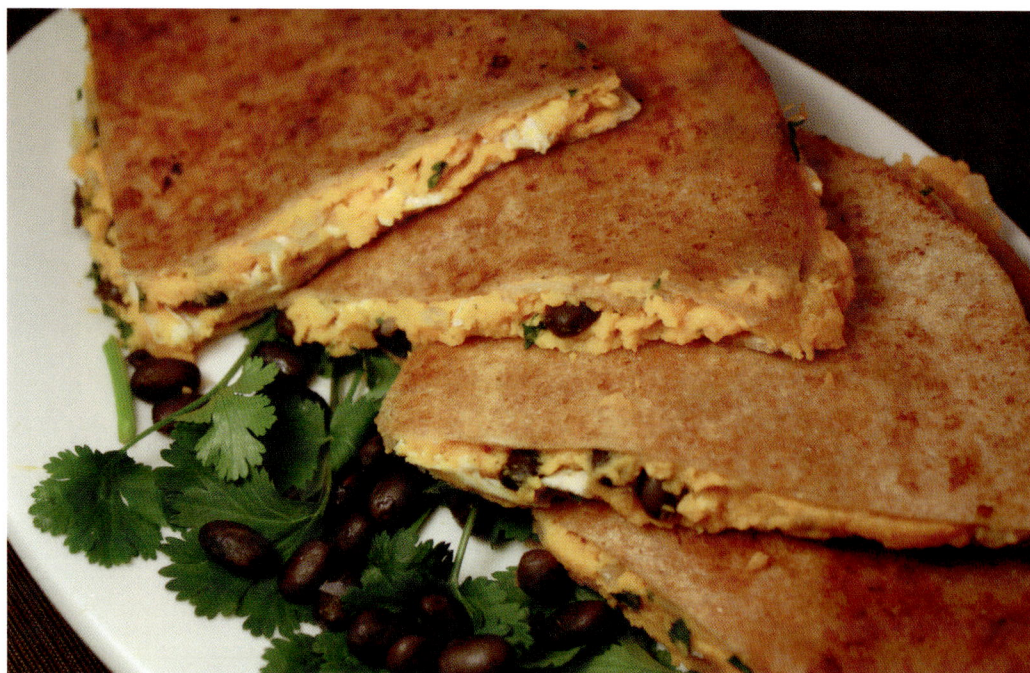

Sweet potatoes are a nice alternative to cheese in these hefty little quesadillas. You can use any combination of onion, green onion, or cilantro that you have on hand - the sweet potatoes are the star here, so the rest is really just window-dressing!

Serves 2

1 pound sweet potato, peeled and cubed
1/3 cup onion, diced
1 Tablespoon olive oil
Four 10-inch whole wheat flour tortillas
1 cup cooked black beans
1-1/2 cups shredded cooked chicken breast
1/4 cup thinly sliced green onions or cilantro leaves
Guacamole to serve (optional) (see Chips and Guacamole in the "Snacks" section)

1. In a pot of boiling water, cook the sweet potato until softened, about 10 minutes. Drain and return to pot, then mash.
2. Meanwhile, sauté the onion and olive oil in a skillet until caramelized. Stir into the potato mash.
3. Spread the potato mash onto two tortillas and scatter with the black beans. Top each with chicken and a few green onions (or cilantro) and a second undressed tortilla. Press to flatten.
4. In a skillet, cook each quesadilla over medium-high heat to heat through, about 4 minutes; flip and cook for about 2 minutes more.
5. Cut into wedges and serve with guacamole.

Roasted Eggplant Dip

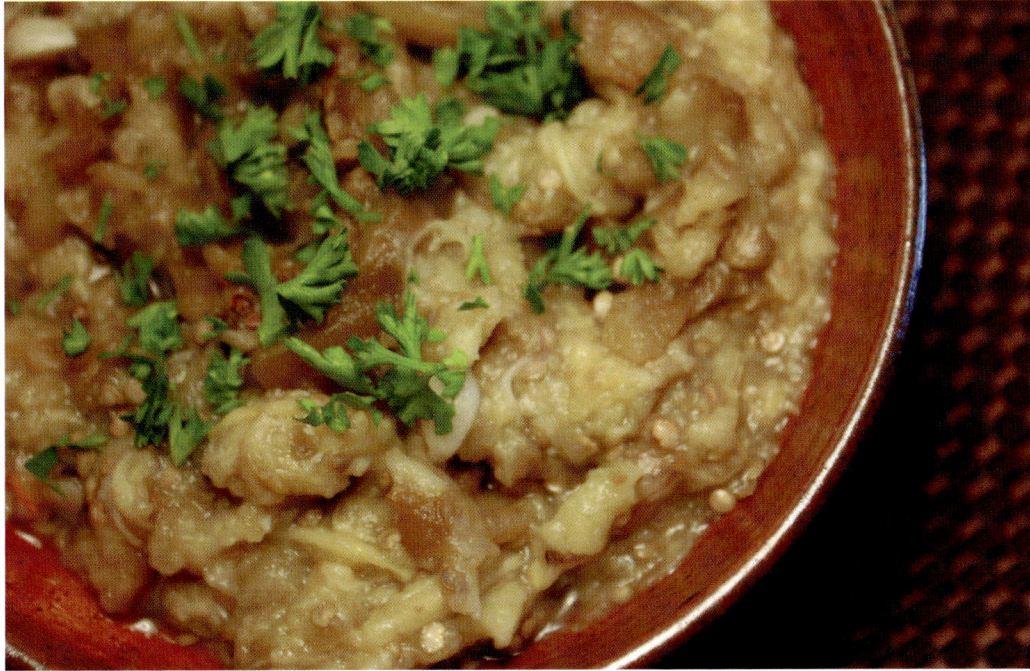

Putting slices of fresh garlic into the roasting eggplant is a great way to add flavor from the inside out. For an Asian twist, you can replace the last tablespoon of olive oil with dark sesame oil and sprinkle the finished slices with sesame seeds. Either way, this is one savory snack dip!

Serves 6

1 large eggplant
6 cloves garlic
Pepper
3 Tablespoons olive oil
Chopped parsley
Crackers or sliced vegetables to serve

1. Preheat the oven to 375 degrees. Oil a baking dish large enough to hold the eggplant.
2. Cut 6 lengthwise slits in the eggplant. Place 2 halves of garlic in each "pocket" of eggplant. Sprinkle pepper in the pockets.
3. Place the eggplant in the baking dish and brush with 2 tablespoon of the oil. Bake for 50 minutes, or until fork tender. Cool.
4. Remove the skin and garlic and place the eggplant in a serving dish. Sprinkle with the remaining tablespoon of olive oil and parsley.
5. Serve with crackers or vegetables.

Broccoli with Fennel & Red Bell Pepper

Attention Francophiles! This dish highlights all things good in French cuisine - fresh produce, beautiful colors, savory aroma, delicious, and effortless. I first sampled this during a visit to Provence, and brought back nearly a suitcase full of herbes de Provence just so I could replicate it at home. Bon appetit!

Serves 4

> 4 Tablespoons olive oil
> 1-1/2 teaspoons fennel seeds
> 2 shallots, chopped
> 1 fresh fennel bulb (about 1 pound), halved lengthwise, thinly sliced cross wise
> 1 large red bell pepper, cut into long strips
> 3 large heads of broccoli, cut into florets (about 7 cups)
> 1 teaspoon herbes de Provence
> 2/3 cup chicken broth
> Salt and pepper (optional)

1. Heat 2 tablespoons olive oil in heavy large skillet over medium heat. Add fennel seeds and stir until toasted, about 3 minutes.
2. Add shallots and sauté until golden, about 3 minutes. Add fennel and bell pepper and sauté until just tender, about 3 minutes.
3. Add broccoli. Drizzle remaining 2 tablespoons oil over vegetables. Crumble the herbs de Provence between fingers into the pot and pour broth over the mixture. Stir to combine.
4. Simmer until broccoli is crisp-tender and liquid evaporates, about 6 minutes.
5. Season with salt and pepper, if desired.

Tip: Herbes de Provence blends can be found online and in the spice section of large supermarkets but you can also mix your own:

> *1 teaspoon dried thyme*
> *1 teaspoon ground rosemary*
> *1 teaspoon summer savory*
> *1/2 teaspoon lavender (optional but traditional)*
> *1 teaspoon marjoram*
> *1 teaspoon dried basil*
> *1/2 teaspoon dried sage*
> *1/2 teaspoon dried oregano*

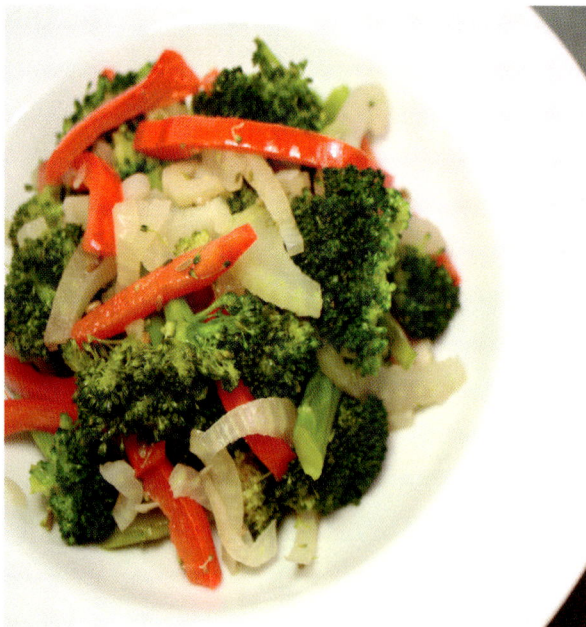

Seared Tuna with Garlic, Tomatoes & Herbs

If there's one recipe from this book that you're going to adopt even after the Elimination Diet is over, this is it. I discovered this dish while vacationing in Alsace, and have since converted many friends and family into tuna-lovers because of it. The original version uses dry white wine in place of the chicken stock, which you can definitely enjoy once you've completed the Challenge Phase.

Serves 4

> 4 tuna steaks, about 1-inch thick (6-7 ounces each)
> Salt and pepper
> 6 Tablespoons olive oil
> 6 cloves garlic, finely chopped
> 4 Tablespoons chicken stock
> 6 ripe tomatoes, seeded and chopped
> 1 Tablespoon dried herbes de Provence
> Fresh basil leaves, to garnish

1. Season the tuna steaks with salt and pepper. Heat a heavy frying pan over high heat until very hot, add the olive oil and swirl to coat. Add the tuna steaks and press down gently, then reduce the heat to medium and cook for 6-8 minutes, turning once, until just slightly pink in the center.
2. Transfer the tuna to a serving plate and cover to keep warm.
3. Add the garlic to the pan and fry for 15-20 seconds, stirring constantly, then pour in the chicken stock and boil until it is reduced by half.
4. Add the tomatoes and dried herbes and cook for 2-3 minutes until the sauce is bubbly.
5. Season with pepper and pour over the fish steaks. Serve, garnished with fresh basil leaves.

Tip: Tuna is often served pink in the middle like beef. If you prefer it cooked through, reduce the heat and cook for an extra few minutes.

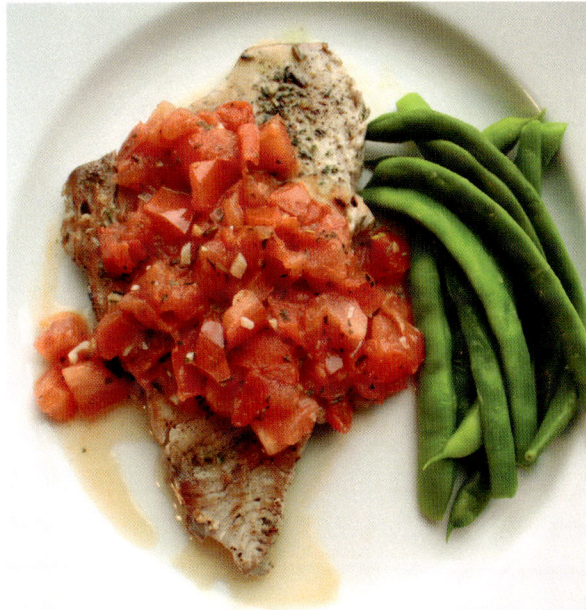

Creamy Mashed Potatoes

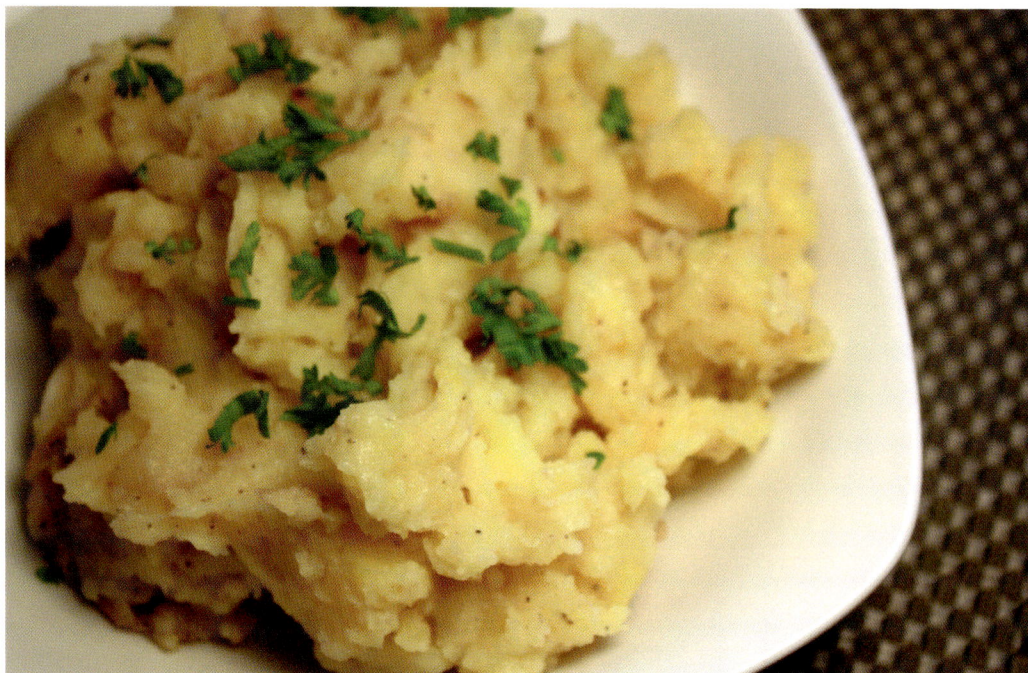

Skins on or skins off? Chunky or smooth? Who knew that one simple dish could ignite such dispute?! However you prefer them, this basic recipe is customizable to meet your own potato mantra and please the masses. If your family likes the skins, the Yukon Gold potato is your best bet since its skins are much thinner than Russets.

Serves 3-4

2-1/2 pounds of potatoes, cut into 1/2 inch cubes
5 to 7 cloves garlic, peeled but not chopped (optional)
1 to 2 Tablespoons olive oil
Salt and pepper to taste
1/2 cup of almond or rice milk (approximately)
Chopped chives or parsley

1. Place potato cubes in a steamer basket and add steamer to a large pot filled with a few cups of water (the water should not rise up enough to touch the potatoes). Cover and bring water to a boil. Steam 4-8 minutes, until potatoes are tender and easily pierced with a fork. Remove steamer from the pot and set aside.
2. If you are making garlic mashed potatoes, preheat the oven to 400 degrees, place garlic on a cookie sheet, and roast it for about 2 minutes. Flip the cloves, and roast for another 2-3 minutes, until lightly browned.
3. Transfer potatoes to a large mixing bowl and add oil, salt and pepper (and roasted garlic, if using). Gently mix, mash, or blend until all ingredients are incorporated.
4. Add the milk a little at a time and blend until the desired consistency is reached. Sprinkle with chives or parsley.

Chicken Teriyaki Meatball Sauté

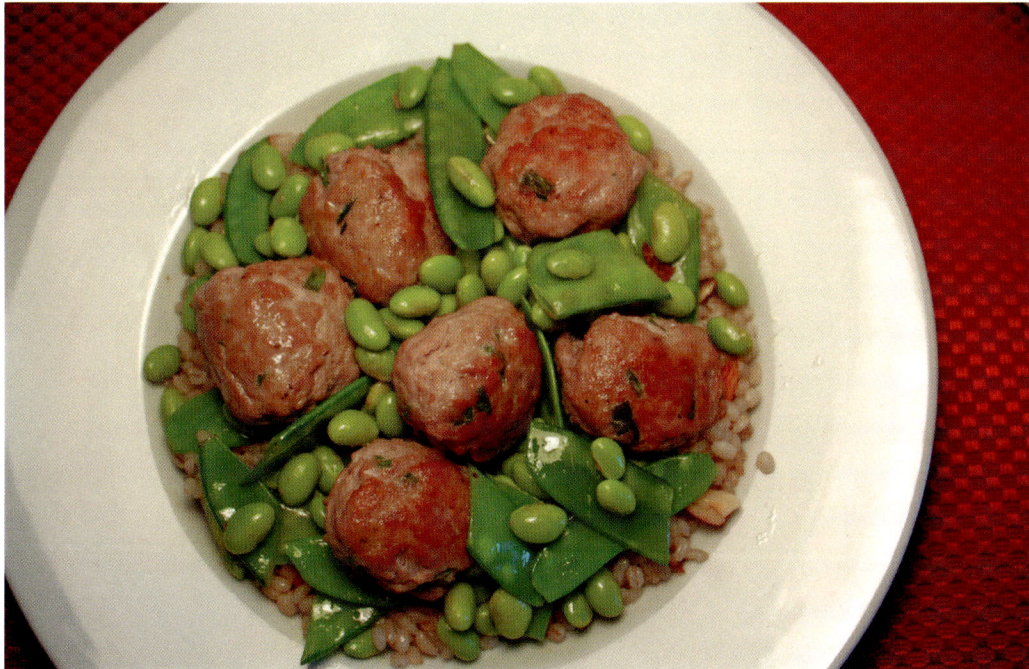

Think meatballs are only Italian food? This fun and unexpected Asian take on the meatball is sure to be a pleasant surprise. One of meatballs' (many) positive qualities is that they freeze exceptionally well, so this recipe is an ideal candidate for doubling or tripling to prepare some quick weeknight dinners in advance.

Adapted from *www.realsimple.com*

Serves 4

- 1-1/4 pounds ground chicken or turkey
- 3 green onions, chopped
- 1/4 to 1/2 teaspoon dried ground ginger, or 2 Tablespoon fresh grated ginger
- 2 Tablespoons olive oil, divided
- 3 cups snow peas, halved crosswise if large (about 1/2 pound)
- 1 cup frozen shelled edamame (soy beans), thawed
- 1/2 cup low-sodium soy sauce
- 1-1/2 to 2 Tablespoons honey or brown rice syrup
- 1-1/2 cups cooked brown rice

1. Combine the chicken, onions, and ginger. Wet hands and shape the mixture into 16 meatballs.
2. Heat 1 tablespoon of the olive oil in a skillet over medium-high heat. Cook the meatballs, turning, until cooked through, 10 to 12 minutes. Transfer to a plate.
3. Heat the remaining oil over medium-high heat in the same skillet. Add the snow peas and edamame. Cook, tossing, for 2 minutes. Return the meatballs to skillet.
4. In a small bowl, combine the soy sauce and honey. Add to the skillet and simmer until slightly thickened, 2 to 3 minutes. Serve over the rice.

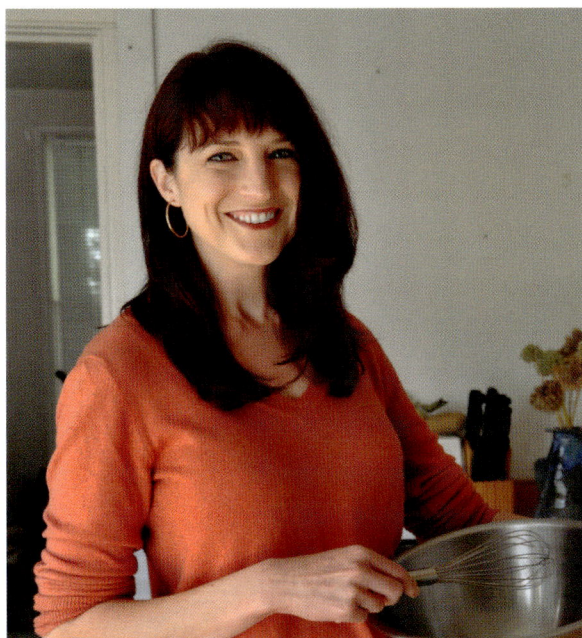

ABOUT THE AUTHOR

Jennifer Vasché Lehner is a passionate home chef and organic vegetable gardener. Jennifer taught herself to cook under the watchful culinary eye of her Italian neighbors while living in Naples, Italy for 2 years during her husband's military service. Since then, she's grown to appreciate and advocate for the beauty and value of simple, quick recipes utilizing fresh produce and quality ingredients.

Jennifer first experienced the Elimination Diet six years ago, and ever since has been providing advice and menu support to friends and family also doing the Elimination Diet - a service that she greatly enjoys and which inspired this book! Jennifer currently resides in Mountain View, CA with her husband, Mike, and son, Luke. She serves as a university research analyst for the University of Washington and in her free time, Jennifer enjoys tending to her vegetable garden, building Lego castles with Luke, and facilitating essential oil educational workshops.

To learn more about the Elimination Diet or Jennifer, please visit www.facebook/eliminationdiet101. She would love to hear from you!